OPCS Classification of Interventions and Procedures, Version 4.7

Volume II

Alphabetical Index

London: TSO

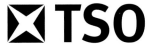

information & publishing solutions

Published by TSO (The Stationery Office) and available from:

Online
www.tsoshop.co.uk

Mail, Telephone, Fax & E-mail
TSO
PO Box 29, Norwich, NR3 1GN
Telephone orders/General enquiries: 0870 600 5522
Fax orders: 0870 600 5533
E-mail: customer.services@tso.co.uk
Textphone: 0870 240 3701

TSO@Blackwell and other Accredited Agents

A Tabular List (volume I) is available separately under ISBN 978 0 11 322990 1
Both volumes can be purchased together at a discounted price, if ordered under
ISBN 978 0 11 322992 5

First published 2014

ISBN 978 0 11 322991 8

Printed in the United Kingdom for The Stationery Office

TABLE OF CONTENTS

INTRODUCTION

Section I: Alphabetical Index of Interventions and Procedures

Welcome to the Alphabetical Index (Volume II) of the OPCS Classification of Interventions and Procedures Version 4.7, April 2014.

The Alphabetical Index (Volume II) is integral to the use of the classification and must be used in conjunction with the primary coding tool – the Tabular List (Volume I). Reference must always be made to the Tabular List in order to select the code which best represents the nature of the intervention performed.

The OPCS-4 is available as an eVersion and replicates the familiar style of the OPCS-4 Tabular List and Alphabetical Index, with the added benefits of a powerful search engine and annotation.

Guide for Use of the Alphabetical Index

The Alphabetical Index must always be used in conjunction with the Tabular List in Volume I.

The Alphabetical Index has four distinct sections, which are:

1. Alphabetical Index of Interventions and Procedures
2. Alphabetical Index of Surgical Eponyms
3. Alphabetical Index of Surgical Abbreviations
4. Alphabetical Index of Common Surgical Suffixes

The Alphabetical Index includes the following abbreviations:

HFQ   However Further Qualified
NEC   Not Elsewhere Classified
NOC   Not Otherwise Classifiable

It also includes abbreviations and curtailed terms:

anast.   = anastomosis
cong.   = congenital
disloc.   = dislocation
endo.   = endoscopic
exam.   = examination
fibreop.   = fibreoptic
gi.   = gastrointestinal
mcp.   = metacarpophalangeal
mtp.   = metatarsophalangeal
prox.   = proximal
recur.   = recurrent
ugi   = upper gastrointestinal

The format of each entry, in general, follows the example below:

ABLATION BRAIN TISSUE STEREOTACTIC:-
ABLATION   = ACTION
BRAIN   = SITE
TISSUE   = SUBSITE
STEREOTACTIC   = ACTION QUALIFIER

Other features

The majority of statements are indexed to the full 4 character code. Additionally, the Alphabetical Index also refers to codes in the format XXX.- e.g. A03.-. This format directs the coder to a variety of qualifying statements at 4-character level in the Tabular List Volume I.

The use of the alpha O carries specific meaning within OPCS-4 because it provides overflow codes to allow interventions to be placed within the correct body system where the chapter has reached capacity. The body system chapter to which the alpha O code relates is represented in the Index by a parenthesis enclosing the chapter prefix. This notation follows the description of the procedure e.g.

O03.- Embolisation Artery Aneurysmal Coil Stent Assisted Transluminal Percutaneous (L)

Endoscopic and minimal access operations that do not have a specific code

The Tabular List of the classification includes a range of categories designated as 'endoscopic' procedures e.g.

M42 Endoscopic extirpation of lesion of bladder

When the classification was constructed it was intended that these categories would be primarily used for operations carried out through existing anatomical passages. However, in the past, some of these categories were also expected to be used for operations carried out using minimal incisions through which rigid or fibreoptic scopes were introduced into body cavities, e.g.

Q37 Endoscopic reversal of female sterilisation

This practice has been maintained in subsequent versions of OPCS-4 and further specific categories have been introduced which differentiate between endoscopic and laparoscopic e.g.

J17.1 Endoscopic ultrasound examination of liver and biopsy of lesion of liver

J09.3 Laparoscopic ultrasound examination of liver NEC

When an endoscopic or minimally invasive procedure (i.e. arthroscopic, thoracoscopic and laparoscopic) is undertaken but no specific code exists to capture this type of approach, dual coding is required. This has the advantage that it can be applied to any existing procedure that may be done via one of these approaches. The preferred form used in the Alphabetical Index is ACCESS MINIMAL.

The primary code is normally that code which is associated with the open form of the procedure. It must be used with maximum clinical detail to identify what was done and on what organ. A second code in the range Y74–Y76 is used to specify the approach. These can be found under the lead terms ACCESS and APPROACH e.g.

Y74 Minimal access to thoracic cavity

When more than one minimally invasive procedure has been undertaken an approach code must be assigned after each open procedure code.

Section II: Alphabetical Index of Surgical Eponyms

The Alphabetical Index of Surgical Eponyms includes a brief description of each intervention, principally to distinguish between those of the same name. If the same operation can be done on different sub sites e.g. parts of the spine, then the eponym is assigned to the unspecified site and reference to the Tabular List suggests allocation to a particular site. Each eponym also has the corresponding OPCS-4 code listed. This index also includes one abbreviation:

(D) = Device.

The device code is assigned to the normal code for insertion or placement. The Tabular List must be consulted for maintenance, removal etc. The use of eponyms is discouraged for coding purposes, and such terms are not used in Section I. They are provided for legacy purposes and have not been updated since OPCS-4.3.

Section III: Alphabetical Index of Surgical Abbreviations

The Alphabetical Index of Surgical Abbreviations includes the description of the abbreviation in addition to the corresponding OPCS-4 code.

Section IV: Alphabetical Index of Common Surgical Suffixes

This section of the Alphabetical Index can be used to rapidly identify the meaning of the more common surgical suffixes.

Training and Advice

The Clinical Classifications Service provides a national service with the primary objective of supporting the NHS.

In addition to developing the OPCS-4 information standard, the Clinical Classifications Service provides expert clinical classifications knowledge on the coding standards in use in the NHS. This covers all aspects of guidance, advice, maintenance, implementation, cross-mapping, coding audit, data quality standards, training and accreditation.

The Classifications and Coding Standards Advisory Service promotes consistent application of the coding standards and use of classifications.

The Clinical Classifications Services is committed to ensuring the NHS clinical coder has access to the highest quality clinical coding training. Our training and accreditation strategy sets a framework to support the NHS and to ensure consistent application of coding standards, giving confidence in the quality of coded clinical data.

For more information on our work:
   http://systems.hscic.gov.uk/data/clinicalcoding

For all queries relating to clinical coding including the Classifications and Coding Standards Advisory Service (helpdesk):
   Email: Information.standards@hscic.gov.uk   Tel: 08451 300 114

For more information on OPCS-4
   http://systems.hscic.gov.uk/data/clinicalcoding/codingstandards/opcs4

To access the online web portal to offer requests for change:
   http://systems.hscic.gov.uk/data/clinicalcoding/codingstandards/opcs4/44submissions

To download the eVersion of the OPCS-4 Tabular List and Index go to the Technology Reference Update Distribution Service (TRUD):
   http://www.uktcregistration.nss.cfh.nhs.uk

Section I

Alphabetical Index
of
Interventions and
Surgical Procedures

A

	Abandoned Operations – refer to Tabular List Introduction
Y50.-	Abdominal Cavity Approach
T45.-	Abdominal Cavity Operations Image Controlled
M52.-	Abdominal Operations Support Bladder Outlet Female NEC
Z31.-	Abdominal Organ site NEC
T31.-	Abdominal Wall Anterior Operations NEC
T31.-	Abdominal Wall Operations NEC
T39.-	Abdominal Wall Posterior Operations
Z53.-	Abdominal Wall site
S02.2	Abdominolipectomy
S02.1	Abdominoplasty
M51.-	Abdominovaginal Operations Support Bladder Outlet Female
	Ablation – see also Destruction
	Ablation – see also Extirpation
	Ablation – see also Resection
K57.4	Ablation Accessory Pathway Transluminal Percutaneous
K62.2	Ablation Atrial Wall Atrial Flutter Transluminal Percutaneous
K57.5	Ablation Atrial Wall Transluminal Percutaneous NEC
K52.-	Ablation Atrioventricular Node
K57.1	Ablation Atrioventricular Node Transluminal Percutaneous
K62.1	Ablation Atrium Left to Vein Pulmonary Transluminal Percutaneous
W35.6	Ablation Bone Lesion Radiofrequency Percutaneous
A03.-	Ablation Brain Tissue Stereotactic
Q16.2	Ablation Endometrium Balloon
Q17.7	Ablation Endometrium Balloon Endoscopic
Q17.6	Ablation Endometrium Microwave Endoscopic
Q16.3	Ablation Endometrium Microwave NEC
Q16.6	Ablation Endometrium Photodynamic
Q16.5	Ablation Endometrium Radiofrequency
Q16.4	Ablation Endometrium Saline Free Circulating
K64.1	Ablation Epicardium Radiofrequency Percutaneous
R04.7	Ablation Fetus Lesion Laser Percutaneous
A03.3	Ablation Globus Pallidus Tissue Stereotactic
K62.3	Ablation Heart Conducting System Atrial Flutter Transluminal Percutaneous
K57.2	Ablation Heart Conducting System Transluminal Percutaneous NEC
K57.7	Ablation Heart Congenital Malformation Transluminal Percutaneous
K16.6	Ablation Heart Septum Chemical Mediated Transluminal Percutaneous
M13.7	Ablation Kidney Lesion Radiofrequency Percutaneous
L88.-	Ablation Leg Vein Varicose
J12.6	Ablation Liver Lesion Chemical Percutaneous

J08.3	Ablation Liver Lesion Microwave Access Minimal
J08.3	Ablation Liver Lesion Microwave Endoscopic
J08.3	Ablation Liver Lesion Microwave Laparoscopic
J12.7	Ablation Liver Lesion Microwave Percutaneous
J03.4	Ablation Liver Lesion Multiple Thermal Open
J12.4	Ablation Liver Lesion Radiofrequency Percutaneous
J03.3	Ablation Liver Lesion Single Thermal Open
J03.3	Ablation Liver Lesion Thermal Open NEC
J12.5	Ablation Liver Lesion Thermal Percutaneous NEC
E59.5	Ablation Lung Lesion Radiofrequency Percutaneous
J66.5	Ablation Pancreas Lesion Chemical Percutaneous
R07.1	Ablation Placental Arteriovenous Anastomosis Laser Endoscopic
R08.1	Ablation Placental Arteriovenous Anastomosis Laser Percutaneous
M67.6	Ablation Prostate Lesion Radiofrequency Endoscopic
M70.7	Ablation Prostate Transurethral Radiofrequency Needle
A03.2	Ablation Thalamus Tissue Stereotactic
X65.5	Ablation Thyroid Radiotherapy Oral Delivery
K57.6	Ablation Ventricular Wall Transluminal Percutaneous
	Access Minimal – refer to Index Introduction
Y75.-	Access Minimal Abdominal
Y76.-	Access Minimal Body Area Other
Y76.-	Access Minimal Body Cavity Other
Y74.-	Access Minimal Thoracic
Z75.6	Acetabulum site
O29.1	Acromioplasty NEC (W)
A70.6	Acupuncture NEC
Y33.1	Acupuncture NOC
E20.-	Adenoid Operations
Z22.5	Adenoid site
E20.1	Adenoidectomy
E20.4	Adenoidectomy Diathermy Suction
F63.3	Adjustment Denture
F15.5	Adjustment Device Orthodontic
C35.-	Adjustment Eye Muscle NEC
F03.3	Adjustment Lip Vermilion Border NEC
C35.-	Adjustment Muscle Eye NEC
F63.3	Adjustment Obturator
	Adjustment Prosthesis – see Prosthesis site
Y15.6	Adjustment Stent NOC
	Adjustment Suture – see Suture site
T70.-	Adjustment Tendon Length
F17.4	Adjustment Tooth Crown Dental
G48.4	Administration Activated Charcoal
	Administration Chemotherapy Neoplasm – see Delivery Chemotherapy Neoplasm
X39.6	Administration Intraocular Therapeutic Substance
X39.-	Administration Therapeutic Substance NEC
X39.5	Administration Transdermal Therapeutic Substance
E95.2	Administration Vaccine Bacillus Calmette-Guerin
X44.-	Administration Vaccine NEC
B25.-	Adrenal Operations NEC

Z14.4	Adrenal site
B23.-	Adrenal Tissue Aberrant Operations
Z14.5	Adrenal Tissue Aberrant site
B22.-	Adrenalectomy
V13.4	Advancement & Bipartition Bone Face & Maxilla
V13.4	Advancement & Bipartition Maxilla & Bone Face
V12.2	Advancement & Remodelling Cranium & Bones Face
V12.1	Advancement & Remodelling Cranium & Orbits
V12.2	Advancement Cranium & Bones Face
V12.1	Advancement Cranium & Orbits
C33.-	Advancement Eye Muscle
V12.2	Advancement Fronto-facial Monobloc
V12.2	Advancement Fronto-facial Split-level
V12.1	Advancement Fronto-orbital
F05.2	Advancement Lip Mucosa NEC
V16.1	Advancement Mandible & Osteotomy
C33.-	Advancement Muscle Eye
S39.-	Allograft Amniotic Membrane
W32.-	Allograft Bone
W32.6	Allograft Bone Bulk
W32.5	Allograft Bone Cancellous Chip
W34.-	Allograft Bone Marrow
W34.6	Allograft Bone Marrow Unrelated Donor Unmatched
Y27.2	Allograft NOC
S37.-	Allograft Skin
W99.1	Allograft Stem Cells Cord Blood to Bone Marrow
Y01.-	Alloreplacement NOC
W34.-	Allotransplantation Bone Marrow
C46.7	Allotransplantation Cornea Limbal Cells
K01.1	Allotransplantation Heart & Lung
K02.1	Allotransplantation Heart NEC
G68.1	Allotransplantation Ileum
G68.-	Allotransplantation Intestine Small NEC
M01.-	Allotransplantation Kidney
K01.1	Allotransplantation Lung & Heart
G26.1	Allotransplantation Stomach
F08.1	Allotransplantation Tooth
F11.1	Alveoplasty Oral
R10.-	Amniocentesis
R10.3	Amnioscopy
R10.-	Amniotic Cavity Operations NEC
Z45.5	Amniotic Membrane site
J39.-	Ampulla Vater Operations Endoscopic Therapeutic NEC
J36.-	Ampulla Vater Operations NEC
Z30.7	Ampulla Vater site
X07.-	Amputation Arm
Q01.1	Amputation Cervix Uteri
P22.-	Amputation Cervix Uteri & Colporrhaphy
P22.-	Amputation Cervix Uteri & Repair Vagina Prolapse
X21.6	Amputation Finger Supernumerary NEC

X10.-	Amputation Foot
X10.1	Amputation Foot Through Ankle
X08.-	Amputation Hand
X09.-	Amputation Leg
N26.-	Amputation Penis
	Amputation Revision – see Amputation site
X12.4	Amputation Stump Bone Revision
X12.4	Amputation Stump Coverage Revision
X12.-	Amputation Stump Operations
X21.5	Amputation Thumb Duplicate
X11.-	Amputation Toe
X27.3	Amputation Toe Supernumerary
X59.1	Anaesthetic Death Preoperative
Y81.-	Anaesthetic Epidural
Y80.-	Anaesthetic General
Y80.-	Anaesthetic Inhalation
Y80.4	Anaesthetic Intravenous
Y82.3	Anaesthetic Local Application NEC
Y82.2	Anaesthetic Local Injection NEC
Y82.-	Anaesthetic Local NEC
C90.-	Anaesthetic Local Ophthalmology Procedures
Y84.-	Anaesthetic NEC
C90.4	Anaesthetic Peribulbar
C90.5	Anaesthetic Retrobulbar
Y81.-	Anaesthetic Spinal
C90.2	Anaesthetic Subconjunctival
C90.3	Anaesthetic Subtenons
C90.1	Anaesthetic Topical Ophthalmology Procedures
X59.-	Anaesthetic without Surgery
H57.-	Anal Sphincter Artificial NEC
Y84.1	Analgesia Gas & Air Labour
E92.4	Analysis Blood Gas
	Anastomosis – see also Bypass
	Anastomosis – see also Connection
	Anastomosis – see also Interposition
	Anastomosis – see also Reanastomosis
	Anastomosis – see also Shunt
L06.-	Anastomosis Aortopulmonary NEC
L07.-	Anastomosis Aortopulmonary Prosthesis Interposition Tube
L50.-	Anastomosis Artery Aortofemoral Emergency
L51.-	Anastomosis Artery Aortofemoral NEC
L50.-	Anastomosis Artery Aortoiliac Emergency
L51.-	Anastomosis Artery Aortoiliac NEC
L34.2	Anastomosis Artery Cerebral
L34.2	Anastomosis Artery Circle Willis
L50.-	Anastomosis Artery Iliofemoral Emergency
L51.-	Anastomosis Artery Iliofemoral NEC
K45.-	Anastomosis Artery Mammary Coronary
L09.-	Anastomosis Artery Pulmonary NEC
L08.-	Anastomosis Artery Subclavian Pulmonary NEC

L07.-	Anastomosis Artery Subclavian Pulmonary Prosthesis Tube Creation
K45.-	Anastomosis Artery Thoracic Coronary
J27.-	Anastomosis Bile Duct & Excision Partial
J46.-	Anastomosis Bile Duct Attention Percutaneous
J30.-	Anastomosis Bile Duct Common
J32.2	Anastomosis Bile Duct Divided End to End
A13.-	Anastomosis Brain Ventricle Component Attention
A14.-	Anastomosis Brain Ventricle NEC
E46.1	Anastomosis Bronchus & Resection Sleeve
H13.-	Anastomosis Caecum
L09.1	Anastomosis Cavopulmonary Superior Bi-directional
H13.-	Anastomosis Colon
H09.-	Anastomosis Colon & Excision Left
H11.-	Anastomosis Colon & Excision NEC
H07.-	Anastomosis Colon & Excision Right
H06.-	Anastomosis Colon & Excision Right Extended
H33.3	Anastomosis Colon & Rectosigmoidectomy
H33.2	Anastomosis Colon Anus & Excision Rectum
H40.4	Anastomosis Colon Anus Trans-sphincteric
H09.2	Anastomosis Colon End to End & Excision Colon Left
H11.1	Anastomosis Colon End to End & Excision NEC
H06.1	Anastomosis Colon End to End & Excision Right Extended
H09.6	Anastomosis Colon End to Side & Excision Colon Left
H11.6	Anastomosis Colon End to Side & Excision NEC
H07.5	Anastomosis Colon End to Side & Excision Right
H06.5	Anastomosis Colon End to Side & Excision Right Extended
H06.2	Anastomosis Colon Ileum & Excision Colon Right Extended
H07.1	Anastomosis Colon Ileum End to End & Excision Colon Right
H11.2	Anastomosis Colon Ileum Side to Side & Excision NEC
H10.2	Anastomosis Colon Rectum & Excision Colon Sigmoid
H09.1	Anastomosis Colon Rectum End to End & Excision Colon Left
H10.-	Anastomosis Colon Sigmoid & Excision
H10.6	Anastomosis Colon Sigmoid End to Side & Excision
H08.-	Anastomosis Colon Transverse & Excision
H08.1	Anastomosis Colon Transverse End to End & Excision
H08.6	Anastomosis Colon Transverse End to Side & Excision
H07.2	Anastomosis Colon Transverse Ileum Side to Side & Excision Colon Right
G58.-	Anastomosis Duodenum & Excision Jejunum
A42.1	Anastomosis Dura Creation
H41.4	Anastomosis Endoanal & Excision Rectum
Q30.3	Anastomosis Fallopian Tube NEC
J19.-	Anastomosis Gall Bladder
J29.-	Anastomosis Hepatic Duct
A36.1	Anastomosis Hypoglossofacial
H04.-	Anastomosis Ileum Anus & Panproctocolectomy
G73.-	Anastomosis Ileum Attention
G72.-	Anastomosis Ileum NEC
H05.-	Anastomosis Ileum Rectum & Excision Colon Total
H08.2	Anastomosis Ileum Rectum & Excision Colon Transverse
H10.1	Anastomosis Ileum Rectum End to End & Excision Colon Sigmoid

G73.-	Anastomosis Intestine Small Attention
G72.-	Anastomosis Intestine Small NEC
G58.-	Anastomosis Jejunum & Excision Jejunum
G61.-	Anastomosis Jejunum NEC
C25.-	Anastomosis Lacrimal Apparatus Nose
A36.2	Anastomosis Nerve Cranial NEC
Y16.2	Anastomosis NOC
G01.-	Anastomosis Oesophagus & Excision Oesophagus & Stomach
G03.-	Anastomosis Oesophagus & Excision Partial
G01.-	Anastomosis Oesophagus & Excision Stomach & Oesophagus
G27.-	Anastomosis Oesophagus & Excision Stomach Total
G02.-	Anastomosis Oesophagus & Excision Total
G06.-	Anastomosis Oesophagus Attention
G06.0	Anastomosis Oesophagus Direct Conversion From
G06.3	Anastomosis Oesophagus Interposition Conversion Direct
G05.-	Anastomosis Oesophagus NEC
J59.-	Anastomosis Pancreatic Duct
H41.1	Anastomosis Peranal & Rectosigmoidectomy
H33.-	Anastomosis Rectum & Excision
H33.-	Anastomosis Rectum & Resection Rectum Anterior
L41.1	Anastomosis Renal Artery End to End & Repair Plastic
G28.-	Anastomosis Stomach & Excision Partial
G31.-	Anastomosis Stomach Duodenum
G58.1	Anastomosis Stomach Ileum & Excision Jejunum Total
G33.-	Anastomosis Stomach Jejunum NEC
G32.-	Anastomosis Stomach Jejunum Transposed
M21.-	Anastomosis Ureter NEC
Q19.1	Anastomosis Uterovaginal
L77.-	Anastomosis Vena Cava
L77.-	Anastomosis Vena Cava Branch
L98.-	Anastomosis Vessel Microvascular
L33.-	Aneurysmectomy Artery Cerebral
L33.-	Aneurysmectomy Artery Circle Willis
K63.-	Angiocardiography Heart
U10.5	Angiocardiography Radionuclide
	Angiography – see also Arteriography
	Angiography – see also Venography
C86.5	Angiography Eye Fluorescein
C87.2	Angiography Retina Indocyanine
U11.7	Angiography Vascular System Magnetic Resonance
L26.-	Angioplasty Aorta Transluminal Percutaneous
L39.1	Angioplasty Artery Axillary Transluminal Percutaneous
L66.5	Angioplasty Artery Balloon Cutting Transluminal Percutaneous
L66.5	Angioplasty Artery Balloon Transluminal Percutaneous
L71.7	Angioplasty Artery Blade Rotary Transluminal Percutaneous
L39.1	Angioplasty Artery Brachial Transluminal Percutaneous
L31.1	Angioplasty Artery Carotid Transluminal Percutaneous
L47.1	Angioplasty Artery Coeliac Transluminal Percutaneous
L69.4	Angioplasty Artery Collateral Systemic to Pulmonary Major Transluminal Percutaneous
K75.3	Angioplasty Artery Coronary & Insertion Stent NEC

K75.1	Angioplasty Artery Coronary Balloon & Insertion Stent Drug-eluting Transluminal Percutaneous
K75.-	Angioplasty Artery Coronary Balloon & Insertion Stent Transluminal Percutaneous
K49.-	Angioplasty Artery Coronary Balloon Transluminal Percutaneous
K49.1	Angioplasty Artery Coronary NEC
K48.3	Angioplasty Artery Coronary Open
K50.1	Angioplasty Artery Coronary Transluminal Percutaneous Laser
L63.1	Angioplasty Artery Femoral Balloon Transluminal Percutaneous
L63.1	Angioplasty Artery Femoral Transluminal Percutaneous
J10.4	Angioplasty Artery Hepatic Transluminal Percutaneous
L54.1	Angioplasty Artery Iliac Transluminal Percutaneous
L47.1	Angioplasty Artery Mesenteric Transluminal Percutaneous
L63.1	Angioplasty Artery Popliteal Balloon Transluminal Percutaneous
L63.1	Angioplasty Artery Popliteal Transluminal Percutaneous
L13.-	Angioplasty Artery Pulmonary Transluminal Percutaneous
L41.6	Angioplasty Artery Renal Patch
L43.1	Angioplasty Artery Renal Transluminal Percutaneous
L39.1	Angioplasty Artery Subclavian Transluminal Percutaneous
L47.1	Angioplasty Artery Suprarenal Transluminal Percutaneous
L71.1	Angioplasty Artery Transluminal Percutaneous
L39.1	Angioplasty Artery Vertebral Transluminal Percutaneous
J10.4	Angioplasty Blood Vessel Liver Transluminal Percutaneous NEC
L97.2	Angioplasty Peroperative
L94.7	Angioplasty Vein Balloon Transluminal Percutaneous NEC
J10.4	Angioplasty Vein Hepatic Transluminal Percutaneous
J11.1	Angioplasty Vein Portal Intrahepatic Transjugular
J10.4	Angioplasty Vein Portal Transluminal Percutaneous
L80.3	Angioplasty Vein Pulmonary Balloon Cutting Transluminal Percutaneous
L80.2	Angioplasty Vein Pulmonary Balloon Transluminal Percutaneous
L99.1	Angioplasty Vein Transluminal Percutaneous NEC
K51.1	Angioscopy Transluminal Percutaneous
L72.3	Angioscopy Transluminal Percutaneous NEC
K34.-	Annuloplasty Heart Valve
H50.-	Anoplasty
G24.-	Antireflux Operations
G24.5	Antireflux Operations & Stomach Operations Plastic
G25.-	Antireflux Operations Revision
E13.3	Antrostomy Intranasal
H56.-	Anus Operations NEC
Z29.2	Anus site
Z96.-	Aorta Abdominal Branch Lateral Other site
Z37.-	Aorta Abdominal Branch Lateral site
L25.4	Aorta Aneurysmal Operations NEC
L28.-	Aorta Aneurysmal Operations Transluminal
L25.-	Aorta Operations Open NEC
L26.-	Aorta Operations Transluminal
K33.-	Aorta Root Operations
Z34.-	Aorta site NEC
Z97.-	Aorta Terminal Branch Other site
Z38.-	Aorta Terminal Branch site
Z95.-	Aorta Thoracic Branch Other site

Z36.-	Aorta Thoracic Branch site
L25.5	Aortic Body Operations
Z40.5	Aortic Body site
L26.4	Aortography
K17.3	Aortopulmonary Reconstruction
L06.1	Aortopulmonary Window Creation
K37.6	Aortoventriculoplasty
K33.6	Aortoventriculoplasty Autograft Valve Pulmonary
X47.1	Apheresis Low-density Lipoprotein
F12.1	Apicectomy Tooth
H01.-	Appendicectomy Emergency
H02.-	Appendicectomy NEC
H14.4	Appendicocaecostomy
H03.3	Appendicostomy
Y51.5	Appendicostomy Approach
H03.-	Appendix Operations NEC
Z28.1	Appendix site
	Application – see also Implantation
	Application – see also Introduction
Y82.3	Application Anaesthetic Local
	Application Band – see Banding site
X49.-	Application Bandage
U33.2	Application Blood Pressure Monitor Ambulatory
F16.6	Application Fluoride Topical
A70.7	Application Nerve Transcutaneous Electrical Stimulator
X48.1	Application Plaster Cast
	Application Ring – see Ringing site
F16.5	Application Sealant Fissure
V18.1	Application Skull Distractor External
X49.5	Application Sling NEC
	Approach – refer to Index Introduction
Y75.4	Approach Abdominal Cavity Hand Assisted Minimal Access
Y75.2	Approach Abdominal Cavity Laparoscopic NEC
Y75.5	Approach Abdominal Cavity Laparoscopic Ultrasonic
Y75.1	Approach Abdominal Cavity Laparoscopically Assisted
Y75.-	Approach Abdominal Cavity Minimal Access
Y50.-	Approach Abdominal Cavity NEC
Y75.3	Approach Abdominal Cavity Robotic Assisted Minimal Access
Y75.3	Approach Abdominal Cavity Robotic Minimal Access
Y51.5	Approach Appendicostomy
Y78.-	Approach Arteriotomy Image Control
Y79.-	Approach Artery
Y79.4	Approach Artery Aortic Transluminal
Y79.2	Approach Artery Brachial Transluminal
Y79.3	Approach Artery Femoral Transluminal
Y79.1	Approach Artery Subclavian Transluminal
Y76.-	Approach Body Area Minimal Access
Y76.3	Approach Body Cavity Endoscopic
Y76.6	Approach Body Cavity Endoscopic Endonasal
Y76.4	Approach Body Cavity Endoscopic Ultrasonic

Y76.-	Approach Body Cavity Minimal Access
Y76.5	Approach Body Cavity Robotic Assisted Minimal Access
Y76.5	Approach Body Cavity Robotic Minimal Access
Y51.4	Approach Colostomy
Y53.3	Approach Control Computed Tomography
Y53.4	Approach Control Fluoroscopic
Y53.-	Approach Control Image
Y53.5	Approach Control Image Intensifier
Y53.7	Approach Control Magnetic Resonance Imaging
Y53.1	Approach Control Radiological
Y53.3	Approach Control Stereotactic
Y53.2	Approach Control Ultrasonic
Y53.6	Approach Control Video
Y47.-	Approach Cranium Contents Burrhole
Y46.7	Approach Cranium Contents Craniectomy
Y46.-	Approach Cranium Contents Open
Y52.3	Approach Cystostomy
Y53.4	Approach Fluoroscopic Control
Y51.-	Approach Gastrointestinal Tract Opening Artificial
Y51.2	Approach Gastrostomy
Y49.4	Approach Heart Transapical
Y49.4	Approach Heart Transventricular
Y51.3	Approach Ileostomy
Y53.-	Approach Image Control
Y53.5	Approach Image Intensifier Control
Y76.7	Approach Joint Arthroscopic
Y50.2	Approach Laparotomy NEC
Y74.5	Approach Mediastinal Cavity Mediastinoscopic
Y71.4	Approach Minimal Access Failed Converted to Open
Y76.1	Approach Nasal Sinus Endoscopic
Y76.2	Approach Nose Endoscopic
Y51.1	Approach Oesophagostomy
Y52.-	Approach Opening Artificial NEC
Y53.-	Approach Percutaneous Control Image
Y71.5	Approach Percutaneous Transluminal Access Failed Converted to Open
Y53.1	Approach Radiological Control
Y48.-	Approach Spine Back
Y48.-	Approach Spine Laminectomy
Y48.4	Approach Spine Pre-sacral Paracoccygeal
Y50.1	Approach Spine Transperitoneal
Y49.2	Approach Spine Transthoracic
Y49.1	Approach Sternotomy Median
Y74.-	Approach Thoracic Cavity Minimal Access
Y74.3	Approach Thoracic Cavity Robotic Assisted Minimal Access
Y74.3	Approach Thoracic Cavity Robotic Minimal Access
Y74.2	Approach Thoracic Cavity Thoracoscopic NEC
Y74.4	Approach Thoracic Cavity Thoracoscopic Video-assisted
Y74.1	Approach Thoracic Cavity Thoracoscopically Assisted
Y49.3	Approach Thoracotomy NEC
Y52.1	Approach Tracheostomy

Y53.2	Approach Ultrasonic Control
Y52.2	Approach Urethrostomy
Y50.3	Approach Vaginal
Y53.6	Approach Video Control
A64.1	Approximation Nerve Peripheral Primary
S02.2	Apronectomy
O31.-	Arm Region Other site NEC (Z)
Z89.-	Arm Region site NEC
E20.3	Arrest Bleeding Adenoid Postoperative Surgical
E05.-	Arrest Bleeding Nose Internal Postoperative Surgical
E05.-	Arrest Bleeding Nose Internal Spontaneous Surgical
	Arrest Bleeding Postoperative Surgical – see also Haemostasis
	Arrest Bleeding Surgical – see also Haemostasis
F36.5	Arrest Bleeding Tonsillar Bed Postoperative Surgical
F16.2	Arrest Bleeding Tooth Socket Postoperative Surgical
K06.1	Arterial Switch Procedure
L04.-	Arterial Tree Pulmonary Operations Open
L39.4	Arteriography Artery Axillary
L39.4	Arteriography Artery Brachial
L31.2	Arteriography Artery Carotid
L35.2	Arteriography Artery Cerebral
L35.2	Arteriography Artery Circle Willis
L47.3	Arteriography Artery Coeliac
K63.-	Arteriography Artery Coronary
L63.4	Arteriography Artery Femoral
J10.7	Arteriography Artery Hepatic
L54.3	Arteriography Artery Iliac
L47.3	Arteriography Artery Mesenteric
L72.1	Arteriography Artery NEC
L72.5	Arteriography Artery Pancreas Stimulated
L63.4	Arteriography Artery Popliteal
L13.3	Arteriography Artery Pulmonary
L43.4	Arteriography Artery Renal
L39.4	Arteriography Artery Subclavian
L47.3	Arteriography Artery Suprarenal
L39.4	Arteriography Artery Vertebral
L02.-	Arteriosus Ductus Patent Operations Open
Y78.-	Arteriotomy Approach Image Control
L75.-	Arteriovenous Operations NEC
L70.5	Artery Aneurysmal Operations NEC
L38.4	Artery Axillary Aneurysmal Operations
L38.-	Artery Axillary Operations Open NEC
L39.-	Artery Axillary Operations Transluminal
Z36.3	Artery Axillary site
O28.1	Artery Basilar site (Z)
L38.4	Artery Brachial Aneurysmal Operations
L38.-	Artery Brachial Operations Open NEC
L39.-	Artery Brachial Operations Transluminal
Z36.4	Artery Brachial site
Z36.7	Artery Brachiocephalic site

Z95.2	Artery Bronchial site
L30.4	Artery Carotid Aneurysmal Operations
Z95.6	Artery Carotid Common site
O12.-	Artery Carotid External Branch site (Z)
Z95.5	Artery Carotid External site
Z95.7	Artery Carotid Internal site
L30.-	Artery Carotid Operations Open NEC
L31.-	Artery Carotid Operations Transluminal
Z36.1	Artery Carotid site NEC
L33.-	Artery Cerebral Aneurysmal Operations
L34.-	Artery Cerebral Operations Open NEC
L35.-	Artery Cerebral Operations Transluminal
Z35.-	Artery Cerebral site
L33.-	Artery Circle Willis Aneurysmal Operations
L34.-	Artery Circle Willis Operations Open NEC
L35.-	Artery Circle Willis Operations Transluminal
Z35.7	Artery Circle Willis site
L46.4	Artery Coeliac Aneurysmal Operations NEC
L46.-	Artery Coeliac Operations Open NEC
L47.-	Artery Coeliac Operations Transluminal
Z37.2	Artery Coeliac site
Z35.-	Artery Communicating site
K48.-	Artery Coronary Operations NEC
K48.-	Artery Coronary Operations Open NEC
K51.-	Artery Coronary Operations Transluminal Diagnostic
K50.-	Artery Coronary Operations Transluminal Therapeutic NEC
Z33.4	Artery Coronary site
Z97.4	Artery Dorsalis Pedis site
L62.4	Artery Femoral Aneurysmal Operations NEC
L62.-	Artery Femoral Operations Open NEC
L63.-	Artery Femoral Operations Transluminal
Z38.-	Artery Femoral site
Z96.1	Artery Gastroduodenal site
Z37.6	Artery Hepatic site
L53.3	Artery Iliac Aneurysmal Operations NEC
Z38.1	Artery Iliac Common site
Z97.5	Artery Iliac External site
Z38.2	Artery Iliac Internal site
L53.-	Artery Iliac Operations Open NEC
L54.-	Artery Iliac Operations Transluminal
Z97.6	Artery Iliac site NEC
Z36.2	Artery Innominate site
Z95.1	Artery Intercostal site
Z96.3	Artery Lumbar site
Z36.6	Artery Mammary Internal site
O12.2	Artery Maxillary site (Z)
L46.4	Artery Mesenteric Aneurysmal Operations NEC
L46.-	Artery Mesenteric Operations Open NEC
L47.-	Artery Mesenteric Operations Transluminal
Z37.-	Artery Mesenteric site

L97.4	Artery Operations NEC
L70.-	Artery Operations Open NEC
L72.-	Artery Operations Transluminal Diagnostic NEC
L71.-	Artery Operations Transluminal Percutaneous NEC
L71.-	Artery Operations Transluminal Therapeutic NEC
Z35.2	Artery Ophthalmic site
Z96.2	Artery Pancreaticoduodenal site
Z97.3	Artery Peroneal site
L62.4	Artery Popliteal Aneurysmal Operations NEC
L62.-	Artery Popliteal Operations Open NEC
L63.-	Artery Popliteal Operations Transluminal
Z38.6	Artery Popliteal site
Z96.5	Artery Pudendal site
L12.-	Artery Pulmonary Operations Open NEC
L13.-	Artery Pulmonary Operations Transluminal
Z40.1	Artery Pulmonary site
Z95.4	Artery Radial site
L42.4	Artery Renal Aneurysmal Operations
L42.-	Artery Renal Operations Open NEC
L43.-	Artery Renal Operations Transluminal
Z37.1	Artery Renal site
Z40.7	Artery site NEC
Z37.7	Artery Splenic site
L38.4	Artery Subclavian Aneurysmal Operations
L38.-	Artery Subclavian Operations Open NEC
L39.-	Artery Subclavian Operations Transluminal
Z36.2	Artery Subclavian site
L46.4	Artery Suprarenal Aneurysmal Operations NEC
L46.-	Artery Suprarenal Operations Open NEC
L47.-	Artery Suprarenal Operations Transluminal
Z37.5	Artery Suprarenal site
O12.1	Artery Temporal Superficial site (Z)
Z96.7	Artery Testicular site
Z97.-	Artery Tibia site
Z95.3	Artery Ulnar site
Z96.6	Artery Uterine site
L38.4	Artery Vertebral Aneurysmal Operations
L38.-	Artery Vertebral Operations Open NEC
L39.-	Artery Vertebral Operations Transluminal
Z36.5	Artery Vertebral site
W62.-	Arthrodesis Joint & Fixation Joint
W61.-	Arthrodesis Joint & Graft Bone Articular NEC
W60.-	Arthrodesis Joint & Graft Bone Extra-articular
W60.-	Arthrodesis Joint & Graft Bone NEC
W64.-	Arthrodesis Joint Conversion NEC
W62.-	Arthrodesis Joint NEC
W63.-	Arthrodesis Joint Revision NEC
W90.2	Arthrography Joint
W78.5	Arthrolysis Joint Elbow NEC
W42.6	Arthrolysis Joint Knee Prosthetic Total

	Arthroplasty – see also Hemiarthroplasty
W57.-	Arthroplasty Joint Excision
X22.-	Arthroplasty Joint Hip Correction Deformity Congenital
W56.-	Arthroplasty Joint Interposition Natural Tissue
W56.-	Arthroplasty Joint Interposition NEC
W55.-	Arthroplasty Joint Interposition Prosthetic
W58.-	Arthroplasty Joint Resurfacing
V20.-	Arthroplasty Joint Temporomandibular
W87.-	Arthroscopy Joint Knee
W88.-	Arthroscopy Joint NEC
W81.4	Arthrotomy Joint NEC
E35.1	Arytenoidectomy Endoscopic
E33.1	Arytenoidectomy External
M48.1	Aspiration Bladder Suprapubic
W36.5	Aspiration Bone Marrow NEC
W36.4	Aspiration Bone Marrow Sternum
A10.2	Aspiration Brain Tissue Abscess
A10.3	Aspiration Brain Tissue Haematoma
A10.4	Aspiration Brain Tissue Lesion NEC
B37.1	Aspiration Breast
E48.4	Aspiration Bronchus Endoscopic NEC
E50.4	Aspiration Bronchus Endoscopic Rigid
E52.2	Aspiration Bronchus NEC
T62.4	Aspiration Bursa
E48.4	Aspiration Carina Endoscopic NEC
E50.4	Aspiration Carina Endoscopic Rigid
V52.5	Aspiration Disc Intervertebral
N15.6	Aspiration Epididymis Lesion
N34.-	Aspiration Epididymis Sperm
Q41.7	Aspiration Fallopian Tube
Y20.4	Aspiration Fine Needle NOC
T61.1	Aspiration Ganglion
Y22.1	Aspiration Haematoma NOC
S47.2	Aspiration Haematoma Skin
N11.5	Aspiration Hydrocele Sac
W90.1	Aspiration Joint
M13.3	Aspiration Kidney Pelvis Percutaneous NEC
M13.3	Aspiration Kidney Percutaneous NEC
C71.3	Aspiration Lens
Y22.2	Aspiration Lesion NOC
J14.2	Aspiration Liver NEC
E48.4	Aspiration Lung Endoscopic NEC
E50.4	Aspiration Lung Endoscopic Rigid
Q51.1	Aspiration Ovary Cyst Transvaginal Ultrasound
J66.4	Aspiration Pancreas Lesion Percutaneous
J67.1	Aspiration Pancreas Lesion Percutaneous Diagnostic
J66.4	Aspiration Pancreas Needle NEC
T12.3	Aspiration Pleural Cavity
P31.3	Aspiration Pouch of Douglas
M70.1	Aspiration Prostate NEC

E48.4	Aspiration Respiratory Tract Lower Endoscopic NEC
E50.4	Aspiration Respiratory Tract Lower Endoscopic Rigid
N34.-	Aspiration Sperm
A48.2	Aspiration Spinal Cord Lesion NEC
A45.6	Aspiration Spinal Cord Lesion Open
E48.4	Aspiration Trachea Endoscopic NEC
E50.4	Aspiration Trachea Endoscopic Rigid
E52.2	Aspiration Trachea NEC
Q11.-	Aspiration Uterus Vacuum Products Conception
U11.6	Assay D-Dimer
U24.2	Assessment Balance
R40.2	Assessment Cervical Length Scanning
R40.1	Assessment Cervix Maternal
E87.4	Assessment Flight
U24.3	Assessment Hearing
X62.-	Assessment NEC
E91.1	Assessment Oximetry
E87.-	Assessment Oxygen
R40.-	Assessment Physiological Maternal
X60.-	Assessment Rehabilitation
X60.4	Assessment Rehabilitation Team Unidisciplinary Specialised
J16.2	Assistance Liver Extracorporeal
K50.4	Atherectomy Artery Coronary Transluminal Percutaneous
L71.7	Atherectomy Artery Transluminal Percutaneous
Z66.1	Atlas site
K05.-	Atrial Inversion Operations Transposition Arteries Great
Z33.6	Atrium Heart site
Z33.1	Atrium Septum site
K22.-	Atrium Wall Operations NEC
	Attachment – see also Reattachment
D05.-	Attachment Auricular Prosthesis
D13.-	Attachment Bone Mastoid Prosthesis Anchored Hearing
E11.2	Attachment Nasal Prosthesis Fixtures First Stage
E11.1	Attachment Nasal Prosthesis Fixtures One Stage NEC
E11.3	Attachment Nasal Prosthesis Fixtures Second Stage
E11.6	Attachment Nasal Prosthesis NEC
C54.-	Attachment Retina Operations Buckling
V41.4	Attachment Spine Correctional Instrument Anterior & Posterior
D05.4	Attention Auricular Fixtures Prosthesis
W05.5	Attention Bone Endoprosthesis
W05.4	Attention Bone Endoprosthesis Massive
D13.4	Attention Bone Mastoid Prosthesis Anchored Fixture Hearing
	Attention Connection – see Connection site
D05.6	Attention Ear External Hearing Implant
D20.5	Attention Ear Middle Hearing Implant
G48.6	Attention Gastric Balloon
G31.6	Attention Gastroduodenostomy
G33.6	Attention Gastroenterostomy NEC
G33.6	Attention Gastrojejunostomy NEC
A54.4	Attention Intrathecal Drug Delivery Device Adjacent Spinal Cord

E31.5	Attention Larynx Voice Box Artificial
T12.5	Attention Pleural Cavity Catheter Tunnelled
T12.5	Attention Pleural Cavity Tube Drain
	Attention Prosthesis – see Prosthesis site
V18.3	Attention Skull Distractor External
V18.4	Attention Skull Distractor Internal
V18.4	Attention Skull Spring
	Attention Stent – see also Placement site Stent
	Attention Stent – see also Prosthesis
Y15.-	Attention Stent NOC
	Attention to Shunt – see Shunt site
	Attention Tube – see Tube
D12.-	Attic Operations
Z20.3	Attic site
D12.7	Atticoantrostomy
D12.2	Atticotomy
U24.-	Audiology Diagnostic
U24.1	Audiometry Pure Tone
A84.4	Auditometry Brain Stem Evoked Response
D08.-	Auditory Canal External Operations NEC
Z20.2	Auditory Canal External site
F11.-	Augmentation Alveolar Ridge
	Augmentation Labour – see Induction Labour
W73.-	Augmentation Ligament Prosthetic
M55.-	Augmentation Urethral Sphincter Female
	Autograft – see also Graft
W31.-	Autograft Bone Cancellous
W31.-	Autograft Bone Cortex
W34.1	Autograft Bone Marrow
W31.6	Autograft Bone Muscle Pedicle
W31.-	Autograft Bone NEC
W31.5	Autograft Bone Vascularised Pedicle
Y27.1	Autograft NOC
W83.7	Autograft Osteochondral Endoscopic
S36.-	Autograft Skin NEC
S35.-	Autograft Skin Split
Y01.1	Autoreplacement NOC
	Autotransplantation – see Transplantation
	Avulsion – see also Destruction
Q02.1	Avulsion Cervix Uteri Lesion
C22.1	Avulsion Eyelid Nerve
L87.4	Avulsion Leg Vein Varicose
S70.1	Avulsion Nail
A60.2	Avulsion Nerve Peripheral
Z66.2	Axis site

B

L74.4	Banding Arteriovenous Fistula
L12.-	Banding Artery Pulmonary
H52.4	Banding Haemorrhoid
J72.5	Banding Spleen
G30.3	Banding Stomach
G30.5	Banding Stomach Maintenance
L01.2	Banding Truncus Arteriosus Persistent
U17.4	Barium Enema
U17.3	Barium Meal
U17.3	Barium Swallow
P03.5	Bartholin Duct Operations
Z44.2	Bartholin Duct site
P03.-	Bartholin Gland Operations
Z44.2	Bartholin Gland site
Z94.1	Bilateral Operations
J41.-	Bile Duct Operations Endoscopic Therapeutic Retrograde NEC
J52.-	Bile Duct Operations NEC
J37.-	Bile Duct Operations Open NEC
J76.-	Bile Duct Operations Percutaneous NEC
J48.-	Bile Duct Operations Percutaneous Other NEC
J49.-	Bile Duct Operations Therapeutic T Tube Track
Z30.-	Bile Duct site
Z30.-	Biliary Tract site
E54.2	Bilobectomy Lung
R37.3	Biometry Fetal
X55.1	Biopsy Abdominal Mass
T31.1	Biopsy Abdominal Wall Anterior
T31.1	Biopsy Abdominal Wall NEC
T39.3	Biopsy Abdominal Wall Posterior
E20.2	Biopsy Adenoid
B25.2	Biopsy Adrenal
J36.2	Biopsy Ampulla Vater
J43.-	Biopsy Ampulla Vater Endoscopic Retrograde
H56.1	Biopsy Anus
L67.1	Biopsy Artery NEC
J44.-	Biopsy Bile Duct Endoscopic Retrograde NEC
J53.1	Biopsy Bile Duct Endoscopic Ultrasonic
J51.1	Biopsy Bile Duct Laparoscopic Ultrasonic
J37.1	Biopsy Bile Duct NEC
J37.1	Biopsy Bile Duct Open

J50.3	Biopsy Bile Duct Percutaneous Transbiliary
J43.-	Biopsy Biliary System Endoscopic Retrograde
M45.-	Biopsy Bladder Endoscopic
M45.-	Biopsy Bladder NEC
M41.4	Biopsy Bladder Open
V13.3	Biopsy Bone Face
W36.5	Biopsy Bone Marrow NEC
W36.-	Biopsy Bone NEC
W36.-	Biopsy Bone Needle Percutaneous
W33.1	Biopsy Bone Open
H25.-	Biopsy Bowel Lower Endoscopic NEC
H25.-	Biopsy Bowel Lower Sigmoidoscope Fibreoptic
H28.-	Biopsy Bowel Lower Sigmoidoscope Rigid
A18.1	Biopsy Brain Endoscopic
A42.2	Biopsy Brain Meninges
A08.-	Biopsy Brain Tissue NEC
A04.-	Biopsy Brain Tissue Open
B32.-	Biopsy Breast
E49.-	Biopsy Bronchus Endoscopic NEC
E51.-	Biopsy Bronchus Endoscopic Rigid
E49.1	Biopsy Bronchus NEC
E47.1	Biopsy Bronchus Open NEC
T62.3	Biopsy Bursa
H22.-	Biopsy Caecum Endoscopic Fibreoptic
H22.-	Biopsy Caecum Endoscopic NEC
H19.1	Biopsy Caecum NEC
H19.1	Biopsy Caecum Open
C11.7	Biopsy Canthus Lesion
E49.1	Biopsy Carina Endoscopic NEC
E51.1	Biopsy Carina Endoscopic Rigid
E44.3	Biopsy Carina Open
Q03.-	Biopsy Cervix Uteri
C84.3	Biopsy Choroid
H22.-	Biopsy Colon Endoscopic Fibreoptic NEC
H22.-	Biopsy Colon Endoscopic NEC
H19.1	Biopsy Colon NEC
H19.1	Biopsy Colon Open
H25.-	Biopsy Colon Sigmoid Endoscopic NEC
H25.-	Biopsy Colon Sigmoid Sigmoidoscope Fibreoptic
H28.-	Biopsy Colon Sigmoid Sigmoidoscope Rigid
H25.-	Biopsy Colon Sigmoidoscope Fibreoptic
H68.1	Biopsy Colonic Pouch Colonoscope
H69.1	Biopsy Colonic Pouch Sigmoidoscope Flexible
H70.1	Biopsy Colonic Pouch Sigmoidoscope Rigid
C43.2	Biopsy Conjunctiva
C51.1	Biopsy Cornea
V05.2	Biopsy Cranium
V52.4	Biopsy Disc Intervertebral NEC
G55.-	Biopsy Duodenum Endoscopic NEC
G55.-	Biopsy Duodenum NEC

G53.1	Biopsy Duodenum Open
G45.-	Biopsy Duodenum Prox. & Examination G.I. Tract Upper Endo. Fibreoptic
G45.-	Biopsy Duodenum Prox. & Examination G.I. Tract Upper Endoscopic NEC
D06.1	Biopsy Ear External
D06.1	Biopsy Ear External Skin
D20.1	Biopsy Ear Middle
D28.1	Biopsy Ear NEC
N15.5	Biopsy Epididymis
C37.3	Biopsy Eye Muscle
C86.1	Biopsy Eye NEC
C10.6	Biopsy Eyebrow Lesion
C22.2	Biopsy Eyelid
C22.2	Biopsy Eyelid Skin
Q39.-	Biopsy Fallopian Tube Access Minimal
Q39.-	Biopsy Fallopian Tube Endoscopic
Q39.-	Biopsy Fallopian Tube NEC
Q34.2	Biopsy Fallopian Tube Open
T57.2	Biopsy Fascia
R02.-	Biopsy Fetus Fetoscopic
R05.1	Biopsy Fetus Percutaneous
J09.-	Biopsy Gall Bladder Access Minimal
J09.-	Biopsy Gall Bladder Endoscopic
J09.-	Biopsy Gall Bladder Laparoscopic
J23.2	Biopsy Gall Bladder NEC
J23.2	Biopsy Gall Bladder Open
J25.1	Biopsy Gall Bladder Percutaneous
J09.-	Biopsy Gall Bladder Peritoneoscope
T61.2	Biopsy Ganglion
G45.-	Biopsy Gastrointestinal Tract Upper Endoscopic Fibreoptic
G45.-	Biopsy Gastrointestinal Tract Upper Endoscopic NEC
G45.-	Biopsy Gastrointestinal Tract Upper NEC
F20.3	Biopsy Gingiva
K23.2	Biopsy Heart NEC
K23.2	Biopsy Heart Wall
H68.3	Biopsy Ileoanal Pouch Colonoscope
H69.3	Biopsy Ileoanal Pouch Sigmoidoscope Flexible
H70.3	Biopsy Ileoanal Pouch Sigmoidoscope Rigid
G80.-	Biopsy Ileum Endoscopic
G78.1	Biopsy Ileum NEC
G78.1	Biopsy Ileum Open
G80.-	Biopsy Intestine Small Endoscopic NEC
G78.1	Biopsy Intestine Small NEC
G78.1	Biopsy Intestine Small Open NEC
T43.-	Biopsy Intra-abdominal Organ Access Minimal
T43.-	Biopsy Intra-abdominal Organ Laparoscopic NEC
T11.-	Biopsy Intrathoracic Organ Access Minimal
T11.-	Biopsy Intrathoracic Organ Thoracoscopic
C64.4	Biopsy Iris
V19.4	Biopsy Jaw NEC
G65.1	Biopsy Jejunum Endoscopic

G67.3	Biopsy Jejunum Mucosa Crosby Capsule
G63.1	Biopsy Jejunum NEC
G63.1	Biopsy Jejunum Open
W88.-	Biopsy Joint Endoscopic NEC
W87.-	Biopsy Joint Knee Endoscopic
W92.1	Biopsy Joint NEC
W69.-	Biopsy Joint Synovial Membrane
M11.1	Biopsy Kidney Endoscopic NEC
M11.2	Biopsy Kidney Endoscopic Retrograde
M13.1	Biopsy Kidney NEC
M08.1	Biopsy Kidney Open
C24.4	Biopsy Lacrimal Gland
C26.3	Biopsy Lacrimal Sac
E36.1	Biopsy Larynx Endoscopic
E37.1	Biopsy Larynx Lesion Microendoscopic Diagnostic
E36.1	Biopsy Larynx NEC
E33.4	Biopsy Larynx Open
C77.3	Biopsy Lens
	Biopsy Lesion – see also Biopsy site
	Biopsy Lesion Excision – see Excision Lesion
Y20.-	Biopsy Lesion NOC
W76.3	Biopsy Ligament
F06.2	Biopsy Lip
F06.2	Biopsy Lip Skin
J09.-	Biopsy Liver Access Minimal
J09.-	Biopsy Liver Endoscopic
J09.-	Biopsy Liver Laparoscopic
J14.1	Biopsy Liver NEC
J05.3	Biopsy Liver Open
J13.2	Biopsy Liver Percutaneous NEC
J09.-	Biopsy Liver Peritoneoscope
J13.1	Biopsy Liver Transjugular
J13.1	Biopsy Liver Transluminal Percutaneous
J13.1	Biopsy Liver Transvascular Percutaneous
J05.3	Biopsy Liver Wedge Open
E49.-	Biopsy Lung Endoscopic NEC
E51.-	Biopsy Lung Endoscopic Rigid
E59.-	Biopsy Lung NEC
T87.-	Biopsy Lymph Node NEC
T91.1	Biopsy Lymph Node Sentinel NEC
V19.4	Biopsy Mandible
D12.3	Biopsy Mastoid
E13.4	Biopsy Maxillary Antrum
E12.8	Biopsy Maxillary Antrum Approach Sublabial
E63.1	Biopsy Mediastinum Endoscopic
E63.1	Biopsy Mediastinum NEC
E61.2	Biopsy Mediastinum Open
T38.3	Biopsy Mesentery Colon NEC
T37.3	Biopsy Mesentery NEC
F42.1	Biopsy Mouth NEC

T81.-	Biopsy Muscle
C37.3	Biopsy Muscle Eye
T81.-	Biopsy Muscle Study
S66.1	Biopsy Nail Bed
E65.1	Biopsy Nasal Cavity Endoscopic
E17.3	Biopsy Nasal Sinus NEC
E25.-	Biopsy Nasopharynx
E25.-	Biopsy Nasopharynx Endoscopic
E27.1	Biopsy Nasopharynx Open
A36.3	Biopsy Nerve Cranial
A73.1	Biopsy Nerve Peripheral
T81.-	Biopsy Neuromuscular Junction
B35.5	Biopsy Nipple
B35.5	Biopsy Nipple Skin
Y20.-	Biopsy NOC
E09.5	Biopsy Nose External
E09.5	Biopsy Nose External Skin
E65.1	Biopsy Nose Internal
E10.1	Biopsy Nose NEC
E03.3	Biopsy Nose Septum
E04.5	Biopsy Nose Turbinate
G45.-	Biopsy Oesophagus & Examination U.G.I. Tract Endoscopic Fibreoptic
G45.-	Biopsy Oesophagus & Examination U.G.I. Tract Endoscopic NEC
G16.-	Biopsy Oesophagus Endoscopic Fibreoptic
G16.-	Biopsy Oesophagus Endoscopic NEC
G16.-	Biopsy Oesophagus NEC
G13.1	Biopsy Oesophagus Open
T36.4	Biopsy Omentum
C06.1	Biopsy Orbit
X55.1	Biopsy Organ Unspecified
Q50.-	Biopsy Ovary Access Minimal
Q50.-	Biopsy Ovary Endoscopic
Q50.-	Biopsy Ovary NEC
Q47.3	Biopsy Ovary Open
F32.1	Biopsy Palate
J45.1	Biopsy Pancreas Endoscopic Retrograde
J74.1	Biopsy Pancreas Endoscopic Ultrasonic
J73.1	Biopsy Pancreas Laparoscopic Ultrasonic
J65.1	Biopsy Pancreas NEC
J65.1	Biopsy Pancreas Open
J67.3	Biopsy Pancreas Percutaneous
J45.1	Biopsy Pancreatic Duct Endoscopic Retrograde
J43.-	Biopsy Pancreatic System Endoscopic Retrograde NEC
J36.2	Biopsy Papilla Vater
B16.2	Biopsy Parathyroid
X55.1	Biopsy Pelvic Mass
N32.1	Biopsy Penis
Y20.5	Biopsy Percutaneous NOC
K71.1	Biopsy Pericardium
T43.1	Biopsy Peritoneal Cavity Access Minimal

T43.1	Biopsy Peritoneal Cavity Endoscopic
T43.1	Biopsy Peritoneum Endoscopic
T41.1	Biopsy Peritoneum NEC
T39.3	Biopsy Peritoneum Posterior
F36.2	Biopsy Peritonsillar Region
E25.-	Biopsy Pharynx Endoscopic
E25.-	Biopsy Pharynx NEC
E27.1	Biopsy Pharynx Open
B04.2	Biopsy Pituitary
R10.5	Biopsy Placenta NEC
R05.1	Biopsy Placenta Percutaneous
T11.-	Biopsy Pleura Access Minimal
T11.-	Biopsy Pleura Endoscopic
T14.-	Biopsy Pleura NEC
T09.2	Biopsy Pleura Open
T11.-	Biopsy Pleural Cavity Access Minimal
T11.-	Biopsy Pleural Cavity Endoscopic
Y20.6	Biopsy Plugged NOC
H68.-	Biopsy Pouch Colonoscope
H69.-	Biopsy Pouch Sigmoidoscope Flexible
H70.-	Biopsy Pouch Sigmoidoscope Rigid
M45.2	Biopsy Prostate Endoscopic
M70.-	Biopsy Prostate NEC
M70.-	Biopsy Prostate Needle
M62.2	Biopsy Prostate Open
G45.1	Biopsy Pylorus NEC
G41.1	Biopsy Pylorus Open
H25.-	Biopsy Rectum Endoscopic NEC
H41.2	Biopsy Rectum Peranal
H25.-	Biopsy Rectum Sigmoidoscope Fibreoptic
H28.-	Biopsy Rectum Sigmoidoscope Rigid
H40.2	Biopsy Rectum Trans-sphincteric
E49.-	Biopsy Respiratory Tract Lower Endoscopic NEC
E51.1	Biopsy Respiratory Tract Lower Endoscopic Rigid
E49.-	Biopsy Respiratory Tract Lower NEC
C84.3	Biopsy Retina
F48.1	Biopsy Salivary Gland
C57.1	Biopsy Sclera
N03.1	Biopsy Scrotum
N03.1	Biopsy Scrotum Skin
N22.4	Biopsy Seminal Vesicle Transrectal Needle
S15.-	Biopsy Skin NEC
S13.-	Biopsy Skin Punch
S14.-	Biopsy Skin Shave
N20.2	Biopsy Spermatic Cord
J36.2	Biopsy Sphincter Oddi
J43.-	Biopsy Sphincter Oddi Endoscopic Retrograde
A51.3	Biopsy Spinal Cord Meninges
A48.1	Biopsy Spinal Cord NEC
A45.4	Biopsy Spinal Cord Open

A45.4	Biopsy Spinal Tract Open
V47.-	Biopsy Spine
J72.3	Biopsy Spleen
Y20.-	Biopsy Stereotactic NOC
G45.1	Biopsy Stomach Endoscopic
G19.-	Biopsy Stomach Gastroscope Rigid
G45.1	Biopsy Stomach NEC
G38.1	Biopsy Stomach Open
S15.-	Biopsy Subcutaneous Tissue
T74.1	Biopsy Tendon NEC
T72.2	Biopsy Tendon Sheath
N13.4	Biopsy Testis
B20.1	Biopsy Thymus
B10.3	Biopsy Thyroglossal Tract
B12.2	Biopsy Thyroid
F24.1	Biopsy Tongue
F36.2	Biopsy Tonsil
E49.-	Biopsy Trachea Endoscopic NEC
E51.-	Biopsy Trachea Endoscopic Rigid
E49.1	Biopsy Trachea NEC
E43.4	Biopsy Trachea Open
T29.4	Biopsy Umbilicus
M30.5	Biopsy Ureter Endoscopic NEC
M25.4	Biopsy Ureter Open
M30.6	Biopsy Ureter Ureteroscope Rigid
M77.-	Biopsy Urethra Endoscopic
M77.-	Biopsy Urethra NEC
M75.1	Biopsy Urethra Open
Q18.1	Biopsy Uterus Endoscopic
Q20.2	Biopsy Uterus NEC
Q09.4	Biopsy Uterus Open
P29.3	Biopsy Vagina
L93.1	Biopsy Vein
K58.4	Biopsy Ventricular Left Transluminal Percutaneous
K58.3	Biopsy Ventricular Right Transluminal Percutaneous
V47.-	Biopsy Vertebra
P09.1	Biopsy Vulva
P09.1	Biopsy Vulva Skin
V13.4	Bipartition Bone Face & Maxilla
V13.4	Bipartition Maxilla & Bone Face
M39.-	Bladder Contents Operations Open NEC
M44.-	Bladder Operations Endoscopic Therapeutic NEC
M43.-	Bladder Operations Increase Capacity Endoscopic
M49.-	Bladder Operations NEC
M41.-	Bladder Operations Open NEC
M48.-	Bladder Operations Other NEC
M56.-	Bladder Outlet Female Operations Endoscopic Therapeutic
M58.-	Bladder Outlet Female Operations NEC
M54.-	Bladder Outlet Female Operations Open NEC
M55.-	Bladder Outlet Female Operations Open Other NEC

M66.-	Bladder Outlet Male Operations Endoscopic Therapeutic NEC
M70.-	Bladder Outlet Male Operations NEC
M64.-	Bladder Outlet Male Operations Open NEC
Z42.-	Bladder site
F13.6	Bleaching Teeth
C65.-	Bleb Operations
C13.-	Blepharoplasty
	Block Nerve – see Nerve Block
W77.-	Blocking Joint
X36.1	Blood Donation
E92.4	Blood Gas Analysis
X32.-	Blood Transfusion Exchange
X32.1	Blood Transfusion Exchange Neonatal
X33.1	Blood Transfusion Intra-arterial
X33.-	Blood Transfusion Intravenous
X33.-	Blood Transfusion NEC
O15.-	Blood Vessel Operations NEC (L)
L97.-	Blood Vessel Operations Other NEC
X36.-	Blood Withdrawal
Z92.-	Body Region site NEC
Z72.-	Bone Arm site NEC
	Bone Autograft – see Autograft Bone
Z63.-	Bone Cranium site
V13.-	Bone Face Operations NEC
Z64.-	Bone Face site NEC
	Bone Flap – see Flap site
Z80.-	Bone Foot site NEC
	Bone Graft – see Graft Bone
Z73.-	Bone Hand site NEC
Z78.-	Bone Leg Lower site NEC
W33.-	Bone Operations Open NEC
Z68.-	Bone Shoulder Girdle site
	Bone site – see also Named Bone site
Z87.1	Bone site NEC
O33.1	Bone Skull Base site (Z)
O33.-	Bone Skull site NEC (Z)
Z72.-	Bone Wrist site NEC
V12.-	Bones Skull Operations NEC
	Bouginage – see also Dilation
M79.1	Bouginage Urethra
H24.-	Bowel Lower Operations Therapeutic Sigmoidoscope Fibreoptic NEC
H62.-	Bowel Operations NEC
Z29.-	Bowel site NEC
Z08.-	Brachial Plexus site
J48.7	Brachytherapy Bile Duct Lesion Percutaneous
Y89.1	Brachytherapy High Dose Rate Treatment
Y89.2	Brachytherapy Pulsed Dose Rate Treatment
A42.-	Brain Meninges Operations NEC
Z05.-	Brain Meninges site
A07.-	Brain Tissue Operations Open

A10.-	Brain Tissue Operations Other
Z01.-	Brain Tissue site
A20.-	Brain Ventricle Operations
A17.-	Brain Ventricle Operations Endoscopic Therapeutic
A16.-	Brain Ventricle Operations Open
Z02.-	Brain Ventricle site
T94.-	Branchial Cleft Operations
	Bravo Ph Capsule – see Insertion Bravo Ph Capsule
B34.-	Breast Duct Operations
B37.-	Breast Operations NEC
B31.-	Breast Operations Plastic NEC
Z15.-	Breast site
R19.-	Breech Delivery Extraction
R20.-	Breech Delivery NEC
E49.-	Bronchoscopy NEC
E51.-	Bronchoscopy Rigid
E48.-	Bronchus Operations Endoscopic NEC
E50.-	Bronchus Operations Endoscopic Rigid
E52.-	Bronchus Operations NEC
E47.-	Bronchus Operations Open NEC
Z24.5	Bronchus site
S01.-	Browlift
Y21.1	Brush Cytology NEC
G45.8	Brushing Gastric NEC
C54.-	Buckling Sclera
W79.2	Bunionectomy
Y47.-	Burr Hole Cranium Contents Approach
V03.6	Burr Hole Cranium Exploratory
T62.-	Bursa Operations
Q32.2	Burying Fimbria Uterus Wall
S03.1	Buttock Lift
M53.1	Buttressing Urethra Vaginal
	Bypass – see also Anastomosis
	Bypass Aorta – see also Replacement Aorta
L16.-	Bypass Aorta
L16.3	Bypass Aorta Anastomosis Artery Axillary Femoral Bilateral
L16.-	Bypass Aorta Emergency
L16.-	Bypass Aorta Extra-anatomic
L20.-	Bypass Aorta Segment Emergency NEC
L21.-	Bypass Aorta Segment NEC
L20.-	Bypass Aorta Segment Prosthesis Emergency NEC
L21.-	Bypass Aorta Segment Prosthesis NEC
	Bypass Artery – see also Replacement Artery
L37.1	Bypass Artery Axillary NEC
L37.1	Bypass Artery Brachial NEC
L29.2	Bypass Artery Carotid Intracranial NEC
L29.3	Bypass Artery Carotid NEC
L45.1	Bypass Artery Coeliac
K46.-	Bypass Artery Coronary
K44.-	Bypass Artery Coronary Graft NEC

L58.-	Bypass Artery Femoral Emergency NEC
L59.-	Bypass Artery Femoral NEC
L50.-	Bypass Artery Iliac Emergency NEC
L50.-	Bypass Artery Iliac Emergency Prosthesis NEC
L51.-	Bypass Artery Iliac NEC
L51.-	Bypass Artery Iliac Prosthesis NEC
L45.1	Bypass Artery Mesenteric
L68.-	Bypass Artery NEC
L58.-	Bypass Artery Popliteal Emergency NEC
L59.-	Bypass Artery Popliteal NEC
L41.2	Bypass Artery Renal
L37.1	Bypass Artery Subclavian NEC
L45.1	Bypass Artery Suprarenal
L37.1	Bypass Artery Vertebral NEC
H13.-	Bypass Caecum
Y73.1	Bypass Cardiopulmonary
H13.-	Bypass Colon
G51.-	Bypass Duodenum
G71.-	Bypass Ileum
G73.-	Bypass Ileum Attention
G73.-	Bypass Intestine Small Attention
G71.-	Bypass Intestine Small NEC
G61.-	Bypass Jejunum
M19.6	Bypass Kidney to Bladder Tunnelled Percutaneous
T89.2	Bypass Lymphatic Duct Obstruction
Y16.3	Bypass NOC
G06.-	Bypass Oesophagus Attention
G05.-	Bypass Oesophagus NEC
L81.2	Bypass Priapism
G31.-	Bypass Stomach Anastomosis Duodenum
G33.-	Bypass Stomach Jejunum NEC
G32.-	Bypass Stomach Jejunum Transposed
L81.-	Bypass Vein NEC

C

M36.1	Caecocystoplasty
H18.-	Caecoscopy Open
H14.-	Caecostomy
H16.2	Caecotomy
H18.-	Caecum Operations Endoscopic Open
H19.-	Caecum Operations Open NEC
Z28.2	Caecum site
R17.-	Caesarean Delivery Elective
R18.-	Caesarean Delivery Emergency
R18.-	Caesarean Delivery NEC
R25.1	Caesarean Hysterectomy
M79.3	Calibration Urethra
A07.6	Callosotomy Complete
A07.7	Callosotomy Partial
C25.1	Canaliculodacryocystorhinostomy
C29.5	Canaliculotomy
	Canalisation – see Recanalisation
L70.4	Cannulation Artery Open
L71.4	Cannulation Artery Transluminal Percutaneous
J08.-	Cannulation Gall Bladder
J08.2	Cannulation Gall Bladder Access Minimal
J08.2	Cannulation Gall Bladder Endoscopic
J07.-	Cannulation Liver
J08.2	Cannulation Liver Access Minimal
J08.2	Cannulation Liver Endoscopic
T89.4	Cannulation Lymphatic Duct
L91.6	Cannulation Vein NEC
L93.4	Cannulation Vein Open
L94.2	Cannulation Vein Transluminal Percutaneous
C15.1	Canthoplasty Medial Ectropion Correction
C11.6	Canthotomy
C11.-	Canthus Operations
Z16.3	Canthus site
Z87.3	Capsule Joint site
Z19.1	Capsule Lens site
C77.1	Capsulectomy
B37.4	Capsulectomy Breast
W81.6	Capsulorrhaphy Joint
B33.2	Capsulotomy Breast
C73.-	Capsulotomy Lens

K76.-	Cardiac Conduit Operations Transluminal
K72.-	Cardiac Defibrillator Subcutaneous
K59.-	Cardiac Defibrillator Transvenous
K61.-	Cardiac Pacemaker System NEC
K60.-	Cardiac Pacemaker System Transvenous
K23.6	Cardiomyoplasty
G09.1	Cardiomyotomy
K66.1	Cardiotachygraphy
K53.-	Cardiotomy
K62.4	Cardioversion Internal Transluminal Percutaneous NEC
X50.-	Cardioversion NEC
K72.-	Cardioverter Defibrillator Other
K59.-	Cardioverter Transvenous
E48.-	Carina Operations Endoscopic NEC
E50.-	Carina Operations Endoscopic Rigid
E44.-	Carina Operations NEC
E44.-	Carina Operations Open
Z24.4	Carina site
L30.5	Carotid Body Operations
Z40.3	Carotid Body site
W02.1	Carpectomy Proximal Row
W02.2	Carpus Operations Metacarpal Support
Z72.-	Carpus site
W83.-	Cartilage Articular Operations Endoscopic Therapeutic NEC
W89.-	Cartilage Articular Operations Endoscopic Therapeutic Other NEC
W82.-	Cartilage Articular Semilunar Operations Endoscopic Therapeutic
W70.-	Cartilage Articular Semilunar Operations NEC
W70.-	Cartilage Articular Semilunar Operations Open
N05.-	Castration Male NEC
A13.-	Catheter Cerebroventricular Shunt Maintenance
A13.-	Catheter Ventricle Brain Shunt Maintenance
A13.-	Catheter Ventriculoperitoneal Shunt Maintenance
A13.-	Catheter Ventriculopleural Shunt Maintenance
A13.-	Catheter Ventriculovascular Shunt Maintenance
O15.3	Catheterisation Arterial Umbilical (L)
M47.-	Catheterisation Bladder Urethral
K65.-	Catheterisation Heart
X41.-	Catheterisation Peritoneal Ambulatory Dialysis
X42.-	Catheterisation Peritoneal Temporary Dialysis
M30.2	Catheterisation Ureter Endoscopic
L91.-	Catheterisation Venous Central
L99.7	Catheterisation Venous Central Peripheral Insertion Transluminal Percutaneous
L94.3	Catheterisation Venous Central Port Subcutaneous Transluminal Percutaneous
O15.2	Catheterisation Venous Umbilical (L)
	Cauterisation – see also Destruction
C66.2	Cauterisation Ciliary Body
Q35.1	Cauterisation Fallopian Tube Bilateral Access Minimal
Q35.1	Cauterisation Fallopian Tube Bilateral Endoscopic
Y13.1	Cauterisation Lesion NOC
Y11.1	Cauterisation NOC

E05.1	Cauterisation Nose Internal
E04.6	Cauterisation Nose Turbinate
S08.-	Cauterisation Skin Lesion & Curettage
S08.-	Cauterisation Subcutaneous Tissue Lesion & Curettage
X20.3	Centralisation Carpus Correction Forearm Deformity Congenital
X23.5	Centralisation Tarsus Correction Leg Deformity Congenital
R21.-	Cephalic Delivery Forceps
R24.-	Cephalic Delivery Normal
R23.-	Cephalic Delivery Vaginal NEC
	Cerclage – see also Wiring
R12.-	Cerclage Uterus Gravid Cervix
R12.2	Cerclage Uterus Gravid Cervix Removal
Q05.1	Cerclage Uterus Non-Gravid Cervix
Z06.5	Cerebrospinal Fluid site
Q55.-	Cervical Smear
Q05.-	Cervix Uteri Operations NEC
Z45.1	Cervix Uteri site
E94.4	Challenge Bronchial
	Change – see also Renewal
X51.-	Change Body Temperature
	Change Pack – see Packing
X48.2	Change Plaster Cast
	Change Tube – see Drainage
	Change Tube – see Tube
C51.2	Chelation Cornea
L71.3	Chemoembolisation Artery Transluminal Percutaneous
X72.-	Chemotherapy Delivery Neoplasm
X73.-	Chemotherapy Delivery Neoplasm Oral
X70.-	Chemotherapy Drugs Neoplasm Procurement Bands 1-5
X71.-	Chemotherapy Drugs Neoplasm Procurement Bands 6-10
X74.-	Chemotherapy Drugs Other
X37.3	Chemotherapy Intramuscular
X35.2	Chemotherapy Intravenous
X38.4	Chemotherapy Subcutaneous
T05.-	Chest Wall Operations NEC
Z52.-	Chest Wall site
J37.-	Cholangiography Access Minimal
J44.-	Cholangiography Endoscopic Retrograde
J37.-	Cholangiography Operative
J50.2	Cholangiography Percutaneous NEC
J50.1	Cholangiography T Tube
J50.5	Cholangiography Transhepatic Percutaneous
J50.4	Cholangiography Transjejunal Percutaneous
J43.-	Cholangiopancreatography Endoscopic Retrograde
U16.2	Cholangiopancreatography Magnetic Resonance
J50.7	Cholangioscopy Transhepatic Percutaneous
J19.1	Cholecystantrostomy
J18.-	Cholecystectomy NEC
J18.-	Cholecystectomy Partial
J18.-	Cholecystectomy Total

X31.1	Cholecystography Intravenous
J19.3	Cholecystojejunostomy
J21.2	Cholecystostomy NEC
J20.2	Cholecystotomy Closure
J21.-	Cholecystotomy NEC
J30.1	Choledochoduodenostomy
J37.4	Choledochoscopy Operative NEC
O19.1	Chondrogenesis Joint Matrix Induced Autologous Endoscopic (W)
W83.4	Chondroplasty Articular Abrasion Endoscopic
W83.5	Chondroplasty Articular Thermal Endoscopic
W89.1	Chondroplasty Endoscopic NEC
E33.3	Chondroplasty Larynx
K38.2	Chordae Tendineae Operations
A44.1	Chordectomy Spinal Cord
E29.5	Chordectomy Vocal Chord & Excision Larynx
E33.2	Chordopexy Vocal Chord
A45.2	Chordotomy Spinal Cord Open NEC
A47.3	Chordotomy Spinal Cord Percutaneous
A45.1	Chordotomy Spinal Cord Stereotactic
A45.2	Chordotomy Spinal Tract Open NEC
A45.1	Chordotomy Spinal Tract Stereotactic
C84.-	Choroid Operations NEC
Z19.4	Choroid site
C67.-	Ciliary Body Operations NEC
	Circle Willis – see Artery Circle Willis
Y73.2	Circulation Extracorporeal NEC
N30.3	Circumcision
A22.3	Cisternography Isotopic
S54.6	Cleansing & Sterilisation Skin Burnt Head
S55.6	Cleansing & Sterilisation Skin Burnt NEC
S54.6	Cleansing & Sterilisation Skin Burnt Neck
S56.6	Cleansing & Sterilisation Skin Head
S57.6	Cleansing & Sterilisation Skin NEC
S56.6	Cleansing & Sterilisation Skin Neck
	Clearance – see also Dissection site Block
E52.2	Clearance Airway
D07.-	Clearance Auditory Canal External
F10.-	Clearance Dental
D15.2	Clearance Ear Middle Suction
E08.8	Clearance Nasal Cavity Suction
X14.-	Clearance Pelvis
X14.1	Clearance Pelvis Total
E89.1	Clearance Respiratory Tract Secretions
E42.8	Clearance Tracheostomy Suction
	Clip – see also Clipping
S41.-	Clip Skin Head Insertion
S42.-	Clip Skin Insertion NEC
S41.-	Clip Skin Neck Insertion
S43.-	Clip Skin Removal
S41.-	Clip Subcutaneous Tissue Head Insertion

S42.-	Clip Subcutaneous Tissue Insertion NEC
S41.-	Clip Subcutaneous Tissue Neck Insertion
S43.-	Clip Subcutaneous Tissue Removal
	Clip Wound – see Clip Skin
	Clipping – see also Clip
L33.2	Clipping Artery Cerebral Aneurysmal
L33.2	Clipping Artery Circle Willis Aneurysmal
Q36.-	Clipping Fallopian Tube Access Minimal NEC
Q35.2	Clipping Fallopian Tube Bilateral Access Minimal
Q35.2	Clipping Fallopian Tube Bilateral Endoscopic
Q27.2	Clipping Fallopian Tube Bilateral Open
Q36.-	Clipping Fallopian Tube Endoscopic NEC
Q28.-	Clipping Fallopian Tube Open NEC
Y07.2	Clipping NOC
P01.1	Clitoridectomy
P01.-	Clitoris Operations
Z44.1	Clitoris site
	Closure – see also Operation site
	Closure – see also Repair
T28.-	Closure Abdomen
T28.8	Closure Abdominal Wall Fistula
L01.4	Closure Aortopulmonary Window
L07.3	Closure Artery Shunt Prosthetic Subclavian Pulmonary
D08.6	Closure Auditory Canal External Blind Sac
T94.2	Closure Branchial Fistula
E47.2	Closure Bronchus Fistula
	Closure Bypass – see Bypass site
C47.-	Closure Cornea
T16.3	Closure Diaphragm Fistula
L02.3	Closure Ductus Arteriosus Patent NEC
G53.2	Closure Duodenum Perforation NEC
G52.-	Closure Duodenum Ulcer NEC
T28.8	Closure Enterocutaneous Fistula
T28.1	Closure Exomphalos
M37.4	Closure Exstrophy
	Closure Fistula – see Closure site Fistula
Y07.3	Closure Fistula NOC
J20.1	Closure Gall Bladder Fistula
G31.5	Closure Gastroduodenostomy
G33.5	Closure Gastroenterostomy NEC
T28.1	Closure Gastroschisis
G78.4	Closure Ileum Perforation
G78.4	Closure Intestine Small Perforation NEC
G63.3	Closure Jejunum Perforation
F03.1	Closure Lip Cleft Primary
F03.2	Closure Lip Cleft Primary Revision
E13.5	Closure Maxillary Antrum Mouth Fistula
E08.6	Closure Nares Anterior Surgical
E03.4	Closure Nose Septum Perforation NEC
G07.-	Closure Oesophagus Fistula

K16.5	Closure Oval Foramen Patent Prosthesis Transluminal Percutaneous
	Closure Perforation – see Closure site Perforation
P13.4	Closure Perineum Female Fistula
T08.4	Closure Pleura Fenestration
T08.2	Closure Pleural Cavity Drainage Open
K34.6	Closure Pulmonary Valve
H33.5	Closure Rectal Stump & Exteriorisation Bowel & Rectosigmoidectomy
H33.5	Closure Rectal Stump & Rectosigmoidectomy & Exteriorisation Bowel
F48.2	Closure Salivary Gland Fistula
Y07.3	Closure Sinus Track NOC
S40.-	Closure Skin NEC
A49.3	Closure Spinal Meningocele
A49.2	Closure Spinal Myelomeningocele
G31.5	Closure Stomach Duodenum Connection
G33.5	Closure Stomach Jejunum Connection
G32.4	Closure Stomach Jejunum Transposed Connection
G36.3	Closure Stomach Opening Abnormal NEC
G36.2	Closure Stomach Perforation NEC
G35.-	Closure Stomach Ulcer NEC
E43.5	Closure Tracheocutaneous Fistula
K34.5	Closure Tricuspid Valve
K38.4	Closure Tunnel Ventricular Aorto-Left
G52.-	Closure Ulcer Duodenal Blood Vessel
M22.3	Closure Ureteric Fistula
M73.3	Closure Urethra Fistula
K38.5	Closure Valsalva Fistula Aortic Sinus
K34.6	Closure Valve Pulmonary
K34.5	Closure Valve Tricuspid
	Coagulation Blood Vessel – see Haemostasis
Q02.3	Coagulation Cervix Uteri Cold
Y10.1	Coblation NOC
Z75.7	Coccyx site
D24.-	Cochlea Operations
Z21.4	Cochlea site
H11.-	Colectomy NEC
H10.-	Colectomy Sigmoid NEC
H05.-	Colectomy Total NEC
H08.-	Colectomy Transverse NEC
	Collar – see Prosthesis
J43.3	Collection Bile Endoscopic Retrograde
J45.-	Collection Pancreatic Juice Endoscopic Retrograde
N34.-	Collection Sperm
M36.3	Colocystoplasty
H21.-	Colon Operations Endoscopic Fibreoptic Therapeutic NEC
H18.-	Colon Operations Endoscopic Open
H21.-	Colon Operations Endoscopic Therapeutic NEC
	Colon Operations NEC – see also Bowel Operations NEC
H30.-	Colon Operations NEC
H19.-	Colon Operations Open NEC
H24.-	Colon Operations Therapeutic Sigmoidoscope Fibreoptic NEC

H24.-	Colon Sigmoid Operations Endoscopic NEC
H62.-	Colon Sigmoid Operations NEC
H27.-	Colon Sigmoid Operations Sigmoidoscope Rigid NEC
H24.-	Colon Sigmoid Operations Therapeutic Sigmoidoscope Fibreoptic NEC
Z28.-	Colon site
H22.-	Colonoscopy NEC
H18.-	Colonoscopy Open
Z29.4	Colorectal site
Y51.4	Colostomy Approach
H33.1	Colostomy End & Excision Rectum Abdominoperineal
H15.-	Colostomy NEC
H15.2	Colostomy Permanent
H32.1	Colostomy Resiting
H15.7	Colostomy Sigmoid Endoscopic Percutaneous
H15.1	Colostomy Temporary
H16.3	Colotomy
P17.-	Colpectomy
P18.-	Colpocleisis
P25.5	Colpoperineorrhaphy
P22.-	Colporrhaphy & Amputation Cervix Uteri
P23.-	Colporrhaphy NEC
Q55.4	Colposcopy Cervix
N34.3	Colposcopy Male
Q55.4	Colposcopy NEC
P27.3	Colposcopy Vagina
M52.3	Colposuspension Bladder Neck NEC
P29.2	Colpotomy NEC
F26.1	Commissurectomy Tongue
X43.-	Compensation Liver Failure
X40.-	Compensation Renal Failure
O15.1	Compression Pseudoaneurysm Duplex Ultrasound Guided (L)
M75.2	Compression Urethra Bulb Male Prosthesis Insertion
Y53.3	Computed Tomography Scan Control Approach
K18.-	Conduit Cardiac Valved
M19.-	Conduit Ileal
C43.-	Conjunctiva Operations NEC
Z18.1	Conjunctiva site
C25.2	Conjunctivodacryocystorhinostomy
	Connection – see also Anastomosis
	Connection – see also Shunt
L06.-	Connection Aortopulmonary NEC
L05.-	Connection Aortopulmonary Prosthesis Interposition Tube Creation
K45.-	Connection Artery Mammary Coronary
L09.-	Connection Artery Pulmonary NEC
L08.-	Connection Artery Subclavian Pulmonary NEC
L07.-	Connection Artery Subclavian Pulmonary Prosthesis Tube Creation
K45.-	Connection Artery Thoracic Coronary
J30.-	Connection Bile Duct Common
A13.-	Connection Brain Ventricle Component Attention
A12.-	Connection Brain Ventricle Creation

A14.-	Connection Brain Ventricle NEC
K17.-	Connection Cavopulmonary Total
J19.-	Connection Gall Bladder
J29.-	Connection Hepatic Duct
G73.-	Connection Ileum Attention
G72.-	Connection Ileum NEC
G73.-	Connection Intestine Small Attention
G72.-	Connection Intestine Small NEC
C25.-	Connection Lacrimal Apparatus Nose
Y16.-	Connection NOC
G06.-	Connection Oesophagus Attention
G05.-	Connection Oesophagus NEC
J59.-	Connection Pancreatic Duct
G31.-	Connection Stomach Duodenum
G33.-	Connection Stomach Jejunum NEC
G32.-	Connection Stomach Jejunum Transposed
M21.-	Connection Ureter NEC
Q19.1	Connection Uterus Vagina
L77.-	Connection Vena Cava
L77.-	Connection Vena Cava Branch
T96.-	Connective Tissue Operations NEC
	Construction – see also Reconstruction
M19.1	Construction Bladder Artificial Ileal
	Construction Conduit – see Conduit site
N28.1	Construction Penis
X15.4	Construction Scrotum
P21.1	Construction Vagina
	Contraceptive Device – see also Operation site
Q12.-	Contraceptive Device Intrauterine
Y97.-	Contrast Radiology
	Control Bleeding – see Arrest Bleeding
	Control Bleeding – see Haemostasis
E89.4	Control Respiration
	Conversion – see Primary Operation site
	Conversion Prosthesis – see Prosthesis site
	Conversion Shunt – see Shunt site
Y15.5	Conversion Stent NOC
X51.2	Cooling Active
C51.-	Cornea Operations NEC
C46.-	Cornea Operations Plastic
C44.-	Cornea Operations Plastic Other
Z18.2	Cornea site
V22.4	Corpectomy Spine Cervical Reconstruction Anterior NEC
V22.4	Corpectomy Spine Cervical Reconstruction Anterior Primary
V23.4	Corpectomy Spine Cervical Reconstruction Anterior Revisional
V25.7	Corpectomy Spine Lumbar Reconstruction Anterior NEC
V25.7	Corpectomy Spine Lumbar Reconstruction Anterior Primary
V26.7	Corpectomy Spine Lumbar Reconstruction Anterior Revisional
V24.4	Corpectomy Spine Thoracic Reconstruction Anterior NEC
V24.4	Corpectomy Spine Thoracic Reconstruction Anterior Primary

V24.5	Corpectomy Spine Thoracic Reconstruction Anterior Revisional
	Correction – see also Repair
X19.-	Correction Arm Upper Deformity Congenital
K05.-	Correction Arteries Great Transposition Atrial Inversion
T02.1	Correction Chest Wall Deformity Pectus
E08.3	Correction Choana Atresia Congenital
W03.3	Correction Claw Toe Total
	Correction Deformity – see also Correction site Deformity
L02.-	Correction Ductus Arteriosus Patent Open
G53.6	Correction Duodenum Malrotation
D03.3	Correction Ear Prominent
C15.4	Correction Ectropion Cicatricial
C15.1	Correction Ectropion NEC
C05.1	Correction Enophthalmos NEC
C15.5	Correction Entropion Cicatricial
C15.2	Correction Entropion NEC
C11.3	Correction Epicanthus
C15.-	Correction Eyelid Deformity
C18.-	Correction Eyelid Ptosis
X21.-	Correction Finger Syndactyly
X27.-	Correction Foot Deformity Congenital Minor
X25.-	Correction Foot Deformity Congenital NEC
X24.-	Correction Foot Deformity Congenital Primary
X24.-	Correction Foot Deformity Congenital Release Foot Joint
X25.2	Correction Foot Deformity Congenital Tarsectomy Wedge
X20.-	Correction Forearm Deformity Congenital
W79.-	Correction Hallux Valgus
W59.5	Correction Hammer Toe
X21.-	Correction Hand Deformity Congenital
X21.2	Correction Hand Mirror
X22.-	Correction Hip Deformity Congenital
T19.3	Correction Hydrocele Infancy
C62.-	Correction Iridodialysis NEC
X23.-	Correction Leg Deformity Congenital
F03.-	Correction Lip Deformity
F03.-	Correction Lip Skin Deformity
E07.1	Correction Nasal Pyriform Aperture Stenosis
X19.2	Correction Obstetric Palsy
G07.3	Correction Oesophagus Atresia Congenital
F29.-	Correction Palate Deformity
T02.-	Correction Pectus Deformity
N28.5	Correction Penis Chordee
K07.-	Correction Pulmonary Venous Connection Anomalous Total
K20.2	Correction Pulmonary Venous Drainage Anomalous Partial
H50.4	Correction Rectum Atresia Congenital Reanastomosis Anal Canal
X19.-	Correction Shoulder Deformity Congenital
K20.1	Correction Sinus Venosus Persistent
V41.-	Correction Spine Deformity Instrumental
V42.-	Correction Spine Deformity NEC
Y15.3	Correction Stent Displacement NOC

C11.4	Correction Telecanthus
X23.2	Correction Tibia Pseudoarthrosis
W03.3	Correction Toe Claw Total
X27.5	Correction Toe Crossed Congenital
X27.4	Correction Toe Fifth Curly
W59.5	Correction Toe Hammer
C15.3	Correction Trichiasis
L01.1	Correction Truncus Arteriosus Persistent
V31.3	Costotransversectomy Disc Intervertebral Thoracic NEC
V32.3	Costotransversectomy Disc Intervertebral Thoracic Revisional
C77.2	Couching Lens
V03.7	Craniectomy Decompressive
V03.9	Craniectomy NEC
V01.7	Craniectomy Sagittal Strip Extended
V01.6	Craniectomy Sagittal Strip Simple
V01.6	Craniectomy Strip
V01.7	Craniectomy Strip with Remodelling Bones Cranial
V01.-	Cranioplasty
V01.5	Cranioplasty Revision NEC
V03.-	Craniotomy
Z63.-	Cranium Bone site
Y47.-	Cranium Contents Approach Burr Hole
Y46.-	Cranium Contents Approach Open
V05.-	Cranium Operations NEC
	Creation – see also Operation site
	Creation Anastomosis – see Anastomosis site
K19.-	Creation Conduit Cardiac Other
K18.-	Creation Conduit Cardiac Valved
C43.6	Creation Conjunctiva Hood
	Creation Connection – see Connection site
	Creation Fistula – see Fistulisation
H57.4	Creation Graciloplasty Sphincter
F63.1	Creation Impression Denture Obturator
F15.1	Creation Impression Orthodontic
F17.2	Creation Impression Tooth Crown Dental
T36.5	Creation Omental Flap
	Creation Reservoir – see Reservoir site
	Creation Shunt – see Shunt site
S63.2	Creation Subcutaneous Storage Pocket & Placement Bone Flap Autologous
S63.2	Creation Subcutaneous Storage Pocket & Placement Tissue Autologous
E42.2	Cricothyroidostomy
M10.4	Cryoablation Kidney Lesion Endoscopic
C72.3	Cryoextraction Lens
	Cryotherapy – see also Destruction
C66.3	Cryotherapy Ciliary Body
Y13.2	Cryotherapy Lesion NOC
A77.-	Cryotherapy Nerve Sympathetic
Y11.2	Cryotherapy NOC
Z79.4	Cuboid site
P31.1	Culdoplasty

P31.4	Culdotomy NEC
Z79.5	Cuneiform site
	Curettage – see also Destruction
S08.-	Curettage & Cauterisation Skin Lesion
S08.-	Curettage & Cauterisation Subcutaneous Tissue Lesion
W09.-	Curettage Bone Lesion
C74.1	Curettage Lens
Y13.3	Curettage Lesion NOC
Y11.3	Curettage NOC
S08.-	Curettage Skin Lesion NEC
S08.-	Curettage Subcutaneous Tissue Lesion NEC
R28.1	Curettage Uterus Delivered
Q10.-	Curettage Uterus NEC
Q10.-	Curettage Uterus Products Conception
H50.3	Cutback Anus Covered
C67.1	Cyclodialysis
F18.1	Cystectomy Dental
M34.-	Cystectomy NEC
M35.-	Cystectomy Partial
J61.1	Cystogastrotomy Pancreas Open
M49.6	Cystography Micturating
U12.7	Cystography Nuclear
M47.8	Cystometry
M34.1	Cystoprostatectomy
M45.-	Cystoscopy
M45.5	Cystoscopy Rigid NEC
	Cystostomy – see also Drainage Bladder
Y52.3	Cystostomy Approach
M49.1	Cystostomy Closure
M38.3	Cystostomy NEC
M34.2	Cystourethrectomy
U12.1	Cystourethrogram Voiding
M37.1	Cystourethroplasty
M45.-	Cystourethroscopy
Y21.1	Cytology Brush NOC
Y21.-	Cytology NOC
E49.-	Cytology Respiratory Tract Lower Brush Endoscopic
E49.-	Cytology Respiratory Tract Lower Brush NEC

D

C25.-	Dacryocystorhinostomy
U06.2	Dacryoscintigraphy
F15.7	Debonding Bracket Orthodontic
W33.2	Debridement Bone Fracture
W33.6	Debridement Bone NEC
C45.7	Debridement Cornea Lesion
W80.-	Debridement Joint
T77.4	Debridement Muscle NEC
Y05.5	Debridement Organ NOC
S54.1	Debridement Skin Burnt Head
S55.1	Debridement Skin Burnt NEC
S54.1	Debridement Skin Burnt Neck
S58.1	Debridement Skin Head Larvae Therapy
S56.1	Debridement Skin Head NEC
S58.2	Debridement Skin Larvae Therapy
S57.1	Debridement Skin NEC
S58.1	Debridement Skin Neck Larvae Therapy
S56.1	Debridement Skin Neck NEC
T96.3	Debridement Soft Tissue NEC
S54.1	Debridement Subcutaneous Tissue Burnt Head
S55.1	Debridement Subcutaneous Tissue Burnt NEC
S54.1	Debridement Subcutaneous Tissue Burnt Neck
S56.1	Debridement Subcutaneous Tissue Head NEC
S57.1	Debridement Subcutaneous Tissue NEC
S56.1	Debridement Subcutaneous Tissue Neck NEC
E42.7	Decannulation Tracheostomy
W18.4	Decompression Bone Fourage
K68.1	Decompression Cardiac Tamponade
V60.-	Decompression Disc Intervertebral Coblation Percutaneous NEC
V60.-	Decompression Disc Intervertebral Coblation Percutaneous Primary
V61.-	Decompression Disc Intervertebral Coblation Percutaneous Revisional
W84.4	Decompression Joint Endoscopic
A32.-	Decompression Nerve Cranial NEC
A73.3	Decompression Nerve Peripheral NEC
C06.3	Decompression Orbit
B04.3	Decompression Pituitary
V22.-	Decompression Posterior Fossa & Spine Cervical Primary
V23.-	Decompression Posterior Fossa & Spine Cervical Revisional
V22.-	Decompression Spine Cervical NEC
V23.-	Decompression Spine Cervical Revisional

V44.-	Decompression Spine Fracture
V25.-	Decompression Spine Lumbar NEC
V26.-	Decompression Spine Lumbar Revisional
V27.-	Decompression Spine NEC
V27.3	Decompression Spine Revisional NEC
V24.-	Decompression Spine Thoracic
V24.3	Decompression Spine Thoracic Revisional
O29.1	Decompression Subacromial (W)
E55.1	Decortication Lung Lesion Open
T07.1	Decortication Pleura
X50.4	Defibrillation Cardiac NEC
X50.4	Defibrillation Ventricular External
E57.3	Deflation Lung Bulla
P07.2	Deinfibulation Vulva
R27.2	Deinfibulation Vulva Delivery Facilitate
C80.3	Delamination Epiretinal Fibrovascular Membrane
R19.-	Delivery Breech Extraction
R20.-	Delivery Breech NEC
R17.-	Delivery Caesarean Elective
R18.-	Delivery Caesarean Emergency
R18.-	Delivery Caesarean NEC
R21.-	Delivery Cephalic Forceps
R24.-	Delivery Cephalic Normal
R23.-	Delivery Cephalic Vaginal NEC
X72.-	Delivery Chemotherapy Neoplasm
X73.-	Delivery Chemotherapy Neoplasm Oral
R27.-	Delivery Facilitated NEC
R25.2	Delivery Facilitated Operations Destructive
R25.-	Delivery NEC
R24.-	Delivery Normal
X65.-	Delivery Radiotherapy
	Delivery Rehabilitation – see Rehabilitation
X65.7	Delivery Therapy Radionuclide NEC
R22.-	Delivery Vacuum
	Demonstration – see Education
L43.6	Denervation Artery Renal Radiofrequency Transluminal Percutaneous
C22.7	Denervation Eyelid Nerve
M08.2	Denervation Kidney Open
M08.2	Denervation Kidney Pelvis Open
A60.6	Denervation Nerve Peripheral
A36.5	Denervation Nerve Trigeminal (v)
V48.-	Denervation Vertebra Spinal Facet Joint
V48.-	Denervation Vertebra Spinal Facet Joint Radiofrequency Controlled
F10.-	Dental Clearance
S60.-	Dermabrasion Skin
S60.5	Dermatoscopy Skin
T56.-	Dermofasciectomy
	Deroofing – see also Marsupialisation
Y06.2	Deroofing Cyst NOC
M04.1	Deroofing Kidney Cyst

M10.3	Deroofing Kidney Cyst Multiple Endoscopic
	Deslough – see Escharotomy
	Deslough – see Removal from Skin Slough
	Destruction – see also Avulsion
	Destruction – see also Extirpation
	Destruction – see also Photodestruction
T31.4	Destruction Abdominal Wall Anterior Lesion
T31.4	Destruction Abdominal Wall Lesion NEC
T39.2	Destruction Abdominal Wall Posterior Lesion
H49.-	Destruction Anus Lesion
D08.1	Destruction Auditory Canal External Lesion
J28.2	Destruction Bile Duct Lesion
M42.-	Destruction Bladder Lesion Endoscopic
M41.1	Destruction Bladder Lesion Open
W09.-	Destruction Bone Lesion
H23.-	Destruction Bowel Lower Lesion Sigmoidoscope Fibreoptic
A38.-	Destruction Brain Meninges Lesion
A17.1	Destruction Brain Ventricle Lesion Endoscopic
B40.-	Destruction Breast Lesion
B40.1	Destruction Breast Lesion Laser Interstitial
E48.-	Destruction Bronchus Lesion Endoscopic NEC
E50.-	Destruction Bronchus Lesion Endoscopic Rigid
E46.4	Destruction Bronchus Lesion Open
E46.-	Destruction Bronchus Partial
H20.-	Destruction Caecum Lesion Endoscopic Fibreoptic
H20.-	Destruction Caecum Lesion Endoscopic NEC
H12.3	Destruction Caecum Lesion NEC
	Destruction Calculus – see Fragmentation
C11.2	Destruction Canthus Lesion
E48.-	Destruction Carina Lesion Endoscopic NEC
E50.-	Destruction Carina Lesion Endoscopic Rigid
Q02.-	Destruction Cervix Uteri Lesion
Y09.-	Destruction Chemical NOC
C66.-	Destruction Ciliary Body
H20.-	Destruction Colon Lesion Endoscopic Fibreoptic
H20.-	Destruction Colon Lesion Endoscopic NEC
H12.3	Destruction Colon Lesion NEC
H23.-	Destruction Colon Lesion Sigmoidoscope Fibreoptic
H23.-	Destruction Colon Sigmoid Lesion Endoscopic NEC
H23.-	Destruction Colon Sigmoid Lesion Sigmoidoscope Fibreoptic
H26.-	Destruction Colon Sigmoid Lesion Sigmoidoscope Rigid
C39.-	Destruction Conjunctiva Lesion
C45.-	Destruction Cornea Lesion
V05.1	Destruction Cranium Lesion
T17.2	Destruction Diaphragm Lesion
V52.-	Destruction Disc Intervertebral
G54.1	Destruction Duodenum Lesion Endoscopic NEC
G50.2	Destruction Duodenum Lesion Open
G43.-	Destruction Duodenum Proximal Lesion & Exam. U.G.I. Tract Endo. Fibreop.
G43.-	Destruction Duodenum Proximal Lesion & Exam. U.G.I. Tract Endo. NEC

D02.2	Destruction Ear External Lesion
D02.2	Destruction Ear External Skin Lesion
D19.2	Destruction Ear Middle Lesion
C12.-	Destruction Eyelid Lesion
C12.-	Destruction Eyelid Skin Lesion
A38.5	Destruction Falx Cerebri Lesion
T53.2	Destruction Fascia Lesion
R06.-	Destruction Fetus
R25.2	Destruction Fetus Facilitate Delivery
Y11.7	Destruction Gamma Wave NOC
A26.3	Destruction Ganglion Trigeminal
G43.-	Destruction Gastrointestinal Tract Upper Lesion Endoscopic Fibreoptic
G42.-	Destruction Gastrointestinal Tract Upper Lesion Endoscopic Fibreoptic Other
G43.-	Destruction Gastrointestinal Tract Upper Lesion Endoscopic NEC
G42.-	Destruction Gastrointestinal Tract Upper Lesion Endoscopic Other NEC
H52.-	Destruction Haemorrhoid
G79.1	Destruction Ileum Lesion Endoscopic
G70.3	Destruction Ileum Lesion Open
G79.1	Destruction Intestine Small Lesion Endoscopic NEC
G70.3	Destruction Intestine Small Lesion Open NEC
C64.3	Destruction Iris Lesion
G64.1	Destruction Jejunum Lesion Endoscopic
G59.2	Destruction Jejunum Lesion Open
M10.1	Destruction Kidney Lesion Endoscopic
M04.3	Destruction Kidney Lesion Open
C24.-	Destruction Lacrimal Gland
C26.2	Destruction Lacrimal Sac Lesion
E35.3	Destruction Larynx Lesion Endoscopic
E34.-	Destruction Larynx Lesion Endoscopic Microtherapeutic
E30.3	Destruction Larynx Lesion Open
Y08.-	Destruction Laser NOC
	Destruction Lesion – see also Destruction site
Y12.-	Destruction Lesion Chemical NOC
Y13.7	Destruction Lesion Microwave NOC
Y13.-	Destruction Lesion NOC
Y13.4	Destruction Lesion Thermal Radiofrequency Controlled NOC
Y13.5	Destruction Lesion Ultrasonic NOC
F02.2	Destruction Lip Lesion
F02.2	Destruction Lip Mucosa Lesion
F02.2	Destruction Lip Skin Lesion
J03.2	Destruction Liver Lesion Open
E48.-	Destruction Lung Lesion Endoscopic NEC
E50.-	Destruction Lung Lesion Endoscopic Rigid
E55.-	Destruction Lung Lesion Open
E62.1	Destruction Mediastinum Lesion Endoscopic
A43.1	Destruction Meninges Skull Base Lesion
A43.2	Destruction Meninges Skull Clivus Lesion
T38.2	Destruction Mesentery Colon Lesion
T37.2	Destruction Mesentery Intestine Small Lesion
Y11.6	Destruction Microwave NOC

F38.-	Destruction Mouth Lesion NEC
T83.1	Destruction Muscle Lesion
S64.-	Destruction Nail Bed
E24.1	Destruction Nasopharynx Lesion Endoscopic
	Destruction Nerve – see also Denervation
A28.8	Destruction Nerve Abducens (vi) Extracranial
A26.2	Destruction Nerve Abducens (vi) NEC
A26.8	Destruction Nerve Accessory (xi) Intracranial
A28.8	Destruction Nerve Accessory (xi) NEC
A28.8	Destruction Nerve Acoustic (viii) Extracranial
A26.5	Destruction Nerve Acoustic (viii) NEC
A28.-	Destruction Nerve Cranial Extracranial
A26.-	Destruction Nerve Cranial Intracranial
A26.4	Destruction Nerve Facial (vii) Intracranial
A28.8	Destruction Nerve Facial (vii) NEC
A28.8	Destruction Nerve Glossopharyngeal (ix) Extracranial
A26.6	Destruction Nerve Glossopharyngeal (ix) NEC
A28.8	Destruction Nerve Hypoglossal (xii) Extracranial
A26.8	Destruction Nerve Hypoglossal (xii) NEC
A28.8	Destruction Nerve Oculomotor (iii) Extracranial
A26.2	Destruction Nerve Oculomotor (iii) NEC
A28.8	Destruction Nerve Optic (ii) Extracranial
A26.1	Destruction Nerve Optic (ii) NEC
A60.-	Destruction Nerve Peripheral
A61.-	Destruction Nerve Peripheral Lesion
A60.4	Destruction Nerve Peripheral Thermal Radiofrequency Controlled
A57.1	Destruction Nerve Root Spinal Lesion
A57.5	Destruction Nerve Root Spinal NEC
A57.3	Destruction Nerve Root Spinal Thermal Radiofrequency Controlled
A76.-	Destruction Nerve Sympathetic Chemical
A79.-	Destruction Nerve Sympathetic NEC
A78.-	Destruction Nerve Sympathetic Thermal Radiofrequency Controlled
A26.3	Destruction Nerve Trigeminal (v) Intracranial
A28.8	Destruction Nerve Trigeminal (v) NEC
A28.8	Destruction Nerve Trochlear (iv) Extracranial
A26.2	Destruction Nerve Trochlear (iv) NEC
A26.7	Destruction Nerve Vagus (x) Intracranial
A27.-	Destruction Nerve Vagus (x) NEC
B35.3	Destruction Nipple Lesion
B35.3	Destruction Nipple Skin Lesion
Y11.-	Destruction NOC
E09.-	Destruction Nose External Lesion
E09.-	Destruction Nose External Skin Lesion
E08.2	Destruction Nose Internal Lesion NEC
G43.-	Destruction Oesophagus Lesion & Exam. U.G.I. Tract Endo. Fibreoptic
G43.-	Destruction Oesophagus Lesion & Exam. U.G.I. Tract Endoscopic NEC
G14.-	Destruction Oesophagus Lesion Endoscopic Fibreoptic
G14.-	Destruction Oesophagus Lesion Endoscopic NEC
G17.-	Destruction Oesophagus Lesion Oesophagoscope Rigid
G04.-	Destruction Oesophagus Lesion Open

T36.3	Destruction Omentum Lesion
C02.2	Destruction Orbit Lesion
X53.-	Destruction Organ Unspecified
Q49.-	Destruction Ovary Lesion Endoscopic
Q44.-	Destruction Ovary Lesion Open
F28.2	Destruction Palate Lesion
J58.3	Destruction Pancreas Lesion
N27.-	Destruction Penis Lesion
N27.-	Destruction Penis Skin Lesion
H49.-	Destruction Perianal Region Lesion
P11.-	Destruction Perineum Female Lesion
N24.8	Destruction Perineum Male Lesion
P11.-	Destruction Perineum Skin Female Lesion
N24.8	Destruction Perineum Skin Male Lesion
T42.2	Destruction Peritoneum Lesion Access Minimal
T42.2	Destruction Peritoneum Lesion Endoscopic
T33.2	Destruction Peritoneum Lesion Open
T39.2	Destruction Peritoneum Posterior Lesion
E24.2	Destruction Pharynx Lesion Endoscopic
H60.1	Destruction Pilonidal Abscess
H60.1	Destruction Pilonidal Cyst
H60.1	Destruction Pilonidal Sinus
B02.-	Destruction Pituitary
T10.1	Destruction Pleura Lesion Endoscopic
T09.1	Destruction Pleura Lesion Open
M67.1	Destruction Prostate Endoscopic Cryotherapy
M67.5	Destruction Prostate Endoscopic Microwave
M67.2	Destruction Prostate Endoscopic NEC
M67.2	Destruction Prostate Endoscopic Ultrasound
M67.-	Destruction Prostate Lesion Endoscopic
M62.1	Destruction Prostate Lesion Open
G43.-	Destruction Pylorus Lesion Endoscopic Fibreoptic
G43.-	Destruction Pylorus Lesion Endoscopic NEC
H23.-	Destruction Rectum Lesion Endoscopic NEC
H34.-	Destruction Rectum Lesion Open
H41.3	Destruction Rectum Lesion Peranal
H23.-	Destruction Rectum Lesion Sigmoidoscope Fibreoptic
H26.-	Destruction Rectum Lesion Sigmoidoscope Rigid
H40.3	Destruction Rectum Lesion Trans-sphincteric
E48.-	Destruction Respiratory Tract Lower Lesion Endoscopic NEC
E50.-	Destruction Respiratory Tract Lower Lesion Endoscopic Rigid
C82.-	Destruction Retina
F45.5	Destruction Salivary Gland Lesion
C53.-	Destruction Sclera Lesion
N01.-	Destruction Scrotum
N01.-	Destruction Scrotum Skin
S10.-	Destruction Skin Lesion Head NEC
S09.-	Destruction Skin Lesion Laser
S11.-	Destruction Skin Lesion NEC
S10.-	Destruction Skin Lesion Neck NEC

A47.1	Destruction Spinal Cord Cervical Substantia Gelatinosa Needle
A44.2	Destruction Spinal Cord Lesion NEC
A51.1	Destruction Spinal Cord Meninges Lesion
A47.-	Destruction Spinal Cord NEC
A44.-	Destruction Spinal Cord Partial
V43.-	Destruction Spine Lesion
A47.2	Destruction Spinothalamic Tract Thermal Radiofrequency Controlled
G43.-	Destruction Stomach Lesion Endoscopic Fibreoptic
G43.-	Destruction Stomach Lesion Endoscopic NEC
G17.-	Destruction Stomach Lesion Gastroscope Rigid
G29.-	Destruction Stomach Lesion Open
S10.-	Destruction Subcutaneous Tissue Lesion Head NEC
S09.-	Destruction Subcutaneous Tissue Lesion Laser
S11.-	Destruction Subcutaneous Tissue Lesion NEC
S10.-	Destruction Subcutaneous Tissue Lesion Neck NEC
C88.-	Destruction Subretinal Lesion
	Destruction Tattoo – see Destruction Skin Lesion
A38.6	Destruction Tentorium Cerebelli Lesion
N07.2	Destruction Testis Lesion
Y11.4	Destruction Thermal Radiofrequency Controlled NOC
F23.2	Destruction Tongue Lesion
F36.1	Destruction Tonsil
E48.-	Destruction Trachea Lesion Endoscopic NEC
E50.-	Destruction Trachea Lesion Endoscopic Rigid
E43.1	Destruction Trachea Lesion Open
A26.3	Destruction Trigeminal Ganglion
Y13.5	Destruction Ultrasonic NOC
T29.3	Destruction Umbilicus Lesion
M29.1	Destruction Ureter Lesion Endoscopic
M32.1	Destruction Ureteric Orifice Lesion Endoscopic
M76.1	Destruction Urethra Lesion Endoscopic
M81.1	Destruction Urethra Meatus Lesion
M76.5	Destruction Urethral Valves Endoscopic
Q17.-	Destruction Uterus Endoscopic
Q52.2	Destruction Uterus Ligament Broad Lesion
P20.-	Destruction Vagina Lesion
C79.-	Destruction Vitreous Body
P06.-	Destruction Vulva Lesion
P06.-	Destruction Vulva Skin Lesion
J07.1	Devascularisation Liver Open
	Device Intrauterine – see Contraceptive Device
X41.-	Dialysis Catheter Ambulatory
X40.-	Dialysis NEC
X40.6	Dialysis Peritoneal Ambulatory Continuous
X40.5	Dialysis Peritoneal Automated
X40.2	Dialysis Peritoneal NEC
X42.1	Dialysis Peritoneal Temporary Catheter Insertion
X40.1	Dialysis Renal
T17.-	Diaphragm Operations NEC
Z53.1	Diaphragm site

	Diathermy – see also Cauterisation
E04.1	Diathermy Nose Turbinate Submucous
O11.-	Digestive Tract Upper Other site (Z)
Z27.-	Digestive Tract Upper site
	Dilatation – see Dilation
H54.-	Dilation Anal Sphincter
H53.2	Dilation Anus Haemorrhoid Forced Manual
L08.6	Dilation Artery Anast. Subclavian Pulmonary Balloon Trans. Percut
L05.4	Dilation Artery Shunt Pulmonary Aorta Balloon Transluminal Percutaneous
L07.4	Dilation Artery Shunt Subclavian Pulmonary Balloon Transluminal Percutaneous
L71.5	Dilation Artery Transluminal Percutaneous
J30.5	Dilation Bile Duct Anastomosis Open
J46.-	Dilation Bile Duct Anastomosis Percutaneous
J76.2	Dilation Bile Duct Balloon Percutaneous
J41.-	Dilation Bile Duct Endoscopic NEC
M58.2	Dilation Bladder Outlet Female
H24.1	Dilation Bowel Lower Sigmoidoscope Fibreoptic
H62.3	Dilation Bowel NEC
H21.1	Dilation Caecum Endoscopic Fibreoptic NEC
H21.1	Dilation Caecum Endoscopic NEC
K76.1	Dilation Cardiac Conduit Balloon Percutaneous Transluminal
Q10.-	Dilation Cervix Uteri & Curettage Uterus NEC
Q11.-	Dilation Cervix Uteri & Evacuation Uterus Products Conception NEC
Q05.2	Dilation Cervix Uteri NEC
H21.1	Dilation Colon Endoscopic Fibreoptic NEC
H21.1	Dilation Colon Endoscopic NEC
H24.1	Dilation Colon Sigmoid Endoscopic NEC
H24.1	Dilation Colon Sigmoid Sigmoidoscope Fibreoptic
H27.1	Dilation Colon Sigmoid Sigmoidoscope Rigid
H24.1	Dilation Colon Sigmoidoscope Fibreoptic
H31.3	Dilation Colorectal Stricture Balloon Image Guided
G54.2	Dilation Duodenum Endoscopic NEC
G44.3	Dilation Duodenum Prox. & Examination U.G.I. Tract Endoscopic Fibreop.
G44.3	Dilation Duodenum Prox. & Examination U.G.I. Tract Endoscopic NEC
Q41.5	Dilation Fallopian Tube NEC
Q34.3	Dilation Fallopian Tube Open
G44.3	Dilation Gastrointestinal Tract Upper Endoscopic Fibreoptic NEC
G44.3	Dilation Gastrointestinal Tract Upper Endoscopic NEC
J29.4	Dilation Hepatic Duct Anastomosis Open
G75.4	Dilation Ileostomy
G79.2	Dilation Ileum Endoscopic
G79.2	Dilation Intestine Small Endoscopic NEC
G64.2	Dilation Jejunum Endoscopic
C27.2	Dilation Lacrimal Duct
C27.2	Dilation Nasolacrimal Duct
E27.5	Dilation Nasopharynx
Y40.-	Dilation NOC
G44.3	Dilation Oesophagus & Examination U.G.I. Tract Endoscopic Fibreoptic
G44.3	Dilation Oesophagus & Examination U.G.I. Tract Endoscopic NEC
G15.-	Dilation Oesophagus Endoscopic Fibreoptic

G15.-	Dilation Oesophagus Endoscopic NEC
G18.-	Dilation Oesophagus Oesophagoscope Rigid
G44.6	Dilation Oesophagus Sphincter Endoscopic Pressure Controlled
G15.5	Dilation Oesophagus Web Endoscopic Fibreoptic
G18.5	Dilation Oesophagus Web Oesophagoscope Rigid
J60.-	Dilation Pancreatic Duct
J42.5	Dilation Pancreatic Duct Endoscopic Retrograde
F55.1	Dilation Parotid Duct
E27.5	Dilation Pharynx
M70.4	Dilation Prostate Balloon
G44.3	Dilation Pylorus Endoscopic Fibreoptic
G44.3	Dilation Pylorus Endoscopic NEC
G40.6	Dilation Pylorus Open
H24.1	Dilation Rectum Endoscopic NEC
H24.1	Dilation Rectum Sigmoidoscope Fibreoptic
H27.1	Dilation Rectum Sigmoidoscope Rigid
F55.-	Dilation Salivary Duct
G44.3	Dilation Stomach Endoscopic Fibreoptic
G44.3	Dilation Stomach Endoscopic NEC
G18.-	Dilation Stomach Gastroscope Rigid
Y40.1	Dilation Stricture NOC
F55.2	Dilation Submandibular Duct
M29.4	Dilation Ureter Endoscopic
M27.7	Dilation Ureter Ureteroscopic
M32.4	Dilation Ureteric Orifice Endoscopic
M76.4	Dilation Urethra Endoscopic
M81.4	Dilation Urethra Meatus
M79.2	Dilation Urethra NEC
P29.5	Dilation Vagina
K35.6	Dilation Valve Pulmonary Transluminal Percutaneous & Perforation
W08.6	Disarticulation Bone NEC
X10.-	Disarticulation Foot
X09.2	Disarticulation Hip
X11.-	Disarticulation Toe
V52.-	Disc Intervertebral Operations NEC
Z99.-	Disc Intervertebral site
C74.2	Discission Cataract
V52.3	Discography Disc Intervertebral
G10.1	Disconnection Vein Azygos
X16.-	Disorders Sex Development Operations
T96.8	Disruption Ganglion Compression
C84.1	Dissection Epiretinal
T85.-	Dissection Lymph Nodes Block
J24.3	Dissolution Gall Bladder Calculus Percutaneous
M43.2	Distension Bladder Hydrostatic Endoscopic
W92.2	Distension Joint
V18.-	Distraction Osteogenesis Skull
V18.-	Distraction Skull
V18.1	Distractor Skull External Application
V18.3	Distractor Skull External Attention

V18.5	Distractor Skull External Removal
V18.4	Distractor Skull Internal Attention
V18.2	Distractor Skull Internal Insertion
V18.6	Distractor Skull Internal Removal
M19.-	Diversion Urinary
M35.1	Diverticulectomy Bladder
	Division – see also Ligation
	Division – see also Transection
	Division Adhesions – see Freeing site Adhesions
W14.-	Division Bone Diaphyseal
V10.-	Division Bone Face
W15.-	Division Bone Foot
W16.-	Division Bone NEC
W12.-	Division Bone Periarticular Angulation
W13.-	Division Bone Periarticular NEC
A07.1	Division Brain Tissue Open
N06.5	Division Cremaster
L02.1	Division Ductus Arteriosus Patent
A51.4	Division Epidural Adhesions Endoscopic
C34.-	Division Eye Tendon Partial
T54.-	Division Fascia
K52.4	Division Heart Accessory Pathway Open
K52.5	Division Heart Conducting System Open NEC
V16.-	Division Jaw NEC
M03.2	Division Kidney Horseshoe Isthmus
E31.3	Division Larynx Stenosis & Insertion Prosthesis
V16.-	Division Mandible
P14.1	Division Muscle Levator Ani & Episiotomy Posterior
T83.2	Division Muscle NEC
G09.3	Division Oesophagus Web
J62.1	Division Pancreas Annular
T41.2	Division Peritoneum Band
A49.1	Division Spinal Filum Terminale Tether
W84.3	Division Synovial Plica Endoscopic
W84.3	Division Synovial Plica Knee Endoscopic
W69.5	Division Synovial Plica Open
C34.-	Division Tendon Eye Partial
Q54.3	Division Uteropelvic Ligament
X36.1	Donation Blood
X46.1	Donation Bone Marrow
X45.2	Donation Heart
X45.1	Donation Kidney
X45.3	Donation Lung Lobe
X45.-	Donation Organ
X46.2	Donation Skin
X46.-	Donation Tissue NEC
Y99.-	Donor Status
Y99.2	Donor Status Live NEC
Y99.5	Donor Status Live Related Matched
Y99.6	Donor Status Live Related Unmatched

	Doppler – see Ultrasound site Doppler
K06.4	Double Switch Procedure
	Drainage – see also Aspiration
	Drainage – see also Evacuation
	Drainage – see also Puncture
T34.3	Drainage Abdominal Abscess Open NEC
T45.3	Drainage Abdominal Abscess Percutaneous Image Controlled NEC
T45.4	Drainage Abdominal Cavity Lesion Percutaneous Image Controlled NEC
T31.5	Drainage Abdominal Wall Anterior
T31.5	Drainage Abdominal Wall NEC
T39.8	Drainage Abdominal Wall Posterior
	Drainage Abscess – see Drainage site Lesion
	Drainage Abscess – see Incision site Lesion
R10.1	Drainage Amniotic Cavity
R07.2	Drainage Amniotic Fluid Twin to Twin Serial Endoscopic
R08.2	Drainage Amniotic Fluid Twin to Twin Serial Percutaneous
X12.5	Drainage Amputation Stump
H03.-	Drainage Appendix
C60.5	Drainage Aqueous Humour
T46.-	Drainage Ascites
D08.3	Drainage Auditory Canal External
P03.4	Drainage Bartholin Gland
J33.-	Drainage Bile Duct NEC
J48.-	Drainage Bile Duct Transhepatic Percutaneous
	Drainage Bladder – see also Catheterisation
M38.1	Drainage Bladder & Urethrostomy Perineal
M38.-	Drainage Bladder Open
M38.2	Drainage Bladder Suprapubic Tube
W18.-	Drainage Bone
A40.-	Drainage Brain Extradural Space
A22.1	Drainage Brain Subarachnoid Space NEC
A41.-	Drainage Brain Subdural Space
A41.2	Drainage Brain Subdural Space Abscess
A05.-	Drainage Brain Tissue Lesion
A20.1	Drainage Brain Ventricle NEC
A16.1	Drainage Brain Ventricle Open NEC
B33.1	Drainage Breast Lesion
H16.1	Drainage Caecum
A53.5	Drainage Cerebrospinal Fluid NEC
T12.4	Drainage Chest Underwater Insertion
H16.1	Drainage Colon
D04.-	Drainage Ear External Lesion
D04.-	Drainage Ear External Skin Lesion
N15.4	Drainage Epididymis
C60.-	Drainage Eye Anterior Chamber Tube
C19.1	Drainage Eyelid Lesion
C19.1	Drainage Eyelid Skin Lesion
Q31.2	Drainage Fallopian Tube
E16.2	Drainage Frontal Sinus NEC
J21.-	Drainage Gall Bladder

J24.1	Drainage Gall Bladder Percutaneous
N11.4	Drainage Hydrocele Sac
H58.1	Drainage Ischiorectal Abscess
W81.3	Drainage Joint
M06.2	Drainage Kidney NEC
M13.2	Drainage Kidney Percutaneous
M16.-	Drainage Kidney Tube
M13.6	Drainage Kidney Tube Insertion Percutaneous
C27.-	Drainage Lacrimal Duct
	Drainage Lesion – see Drainage site Lesion
J05.1	Drainage Liver Open
J12.1	Drainage Liver Percutaneous
E59.4	Drainage Lung
T88.-	Drainage Lymph Node Lesion
E12.2	Drainage Maxillary Antrum Approach Sublabial
E13.1	Drainage Maxillary Antrum NEC
E61.3	Drainage Mediastinum Open
C27.-	Drainage Nasolacrimal Duct
Y22.-	Drainage NOC
G09.4	Drainage Oesophagus
C06.2	Drainage Orbit
Q49.3	Drainage Ovary Cyst Access Minimal
Q49.3	Drainage Ovary Cyst Endoscopic
Q47.4	Drainage Ovary Cyst Open
J42.4	Drainage Pancreas Lesion Endoscopic Retrograde
J61.-	Drainage Pancreas Lesion Open
J66.-	Drainage Pancreas Lesion Percutaneous
J60.-	Drainage Pancreatic Duct
E27.2	Drainage Parapharyngeal Abscess
M83.1	Drainage Paravesical Abscess
T34.2	Drainage Pelvic Abscess Open
T45.2	Drainage Pelvic Abscess Percutaneous Image Controlled
N32.2	Drainage Penis
H58.2	Drainage Perianal Abscess
K68.-	Drainage Pericardium
K77.-	Drainage Pericardium Transluminal
H16.1	Drainage Pericolonic Tissue
H58.-	Drainage Perineal Region Through
P13.1	Drainage Perineum Female
P13.1	Drainage Perineum Skin Female
G09.4	Drainage Perioesophageal Tissue
H58.3	Drainage Perirectal Abscess
T46.-	Drainage Peritoneal Cavity NEC
T34.-	Drainage Peritoneum Open
F36.3	Drainage Peritonsillar Region Abscess
H60.3	Drainage Pilonidal Abscess
H60.3	Drainage Pilonidal Cyst
H60.3	Drainage Pilonidal Sinus
T12.1	Drainage Pleura Lesion NEC
T12.4	Drainage Pleural Cavity Catheter Tunnelled Insertion

T12.-	Drainage Pleural Cavity NEC
T08.-	Drainage Pleural Cavity Open
T12.4	Drainage Pleural Cavity Tube Insertion
P31.2	Drainage Pouch Douglas
M67.3	Drainage Prostate Endoscopic
	Drainage Removal – see also Removal from site
E27.2	Drainage Retropharyngeal Abscess
C55.1	Drainage Sclera Lesion
N03.2	Drainage Scrotum
S47.-	Drainage Skin Lesion
N20.3	Drainage Spermatic Cord
E15.1	Drainage Sphenoid Sinus
A53.-	Drainage Spinal Canal
S47.-	Drainage Subcutaneous Tissue Lesion
T34.1	Drainage Subphrenic Abscess Open
T45.1	Drainage Subphrenic Abscess Percutaneous Image Controlled
C84.5	Drainage Subretinal Fluid Through Retina
C55.3	Drainage Subretinal Fluid Through Sclera
N13.1	Drainage Testis
F16.1	Drainage Tooth Alveolus Abscess
M28.-	Drainage Ureter Calculus Endoscopic
P09.2	Drainage Vulva Lesion
S54.-	Dressing Skin Burnt Head
S55.-	Dressing Skin Burnt NEC
S54.-	Dressing Skin Burnt Neck
S56.-	Dressing Skin Head NEC
S57.-	Dressing Skin NEC
S56.-	Dressing Skin Neck NEC
S54.-	Dressing Subcutaneous Tissue Burnt Head
S55.-	Dressing Subcutaneous Tissue Burnt NEC
S54.-	Dressing Subcutaneous Tissue Burnt Neck
S56.-	Dressing Subcutaneous Tissue Head NEC
S57.-	Dressing Subcutaneous Tissue NEC
S56.-	Dressing Subcutaneous Tissue Neck NEC
W36.3	Drilling Bone Diagnostic
W35.4	Drilling Bone Therapeutic NEC
W71.1	Drilling Cartilage Articular
W83.1	Drilling Cartilage Articular Lesion Endoscopic
W84.5	Drilling Epiphysis Cartilage Articular Repair Endoscopic
Y33.2	Drilling NOC
Q49.4	Drilling Ovary Endoscopic
L03.-	Ductus Arteriosus Patent Operations Transluminal
G49.-	Duodenectomy
G51.4	Duodeno-colostomy
G51.2	Duodeno-duodenostomy
G51.3	Duodeno-jejunostomy
G55.-	Duodenoscopy
G53.5	Duodenotomy NEC
G54.-	Duodenum Operations Endoscopic Therapeutic NEC
G57.-	Duodenum Operations NEC

G53.-	Duodenum Operations Open NEC
Z27.4	Duodenum site
G52.-	Duodenum Ulcer Operations
Q41.3	Dye Test Fallopian Tube

E

D06.-	Ear External Operations NEC
D03.-	Ear External Operations Plastic
Z20.1	Ear External site
D06.-	Ear External Skin Operations NEC
D03.-	Ear External Skin Operations Plastic
Z20.1	Ear External Skin site
D23.-	Ear Inner Operations NEC
Z21.6	Ear Inner site
D20.-	Ear Middle Operations NEC
Z21.2	Ear Middle site
D28.-	Ear Operations NEC
D17.-	Ear Ossicle Operations NEC
Z21.1	Ear Ossicle site
Z20.-	Ear Outer site
Z21.-	Ear site NEC
Z20.4	Eardrum site
Y70.-	Early Operations NOC
U20.-	Echocardiography Diagnostic
U20.3	Echocardiography Intravascular
U20.1	Echocardiography NEC
K58.5	Echocardiography Transluminal
U20.2	Echocardiography Transoesophageal
U20.1	Echocardiography Transthoracic
E97.1	Education Inhaler
E97.1	Education Nebuliser
E97.2	Education Peak Flow Technique
E97.-	Education Respiratory
E97.3	Education Respiratory Health Self-management
E97.1	Education Therapy Inhaled
U36.4	Elastography Ultrasound
A70.5	Electroacupuncture
U19.-	Electrocardiography Diagnostic
Y17.1	Electrocauterisation Lesion NOC
Y10.2	Electrocauterisation NOC
Y12.3	Electrochemotherapy Lesion NOC
D24.5	Electrocochleography Transtympanic
A83.-	Electroconvulsive Therapy
S10.5	Electrodessication Skin Lesion Head
S11.5	Electrodessication Skin Lesion NEC
S10.5	Electrodessication Skin Lesion Neck

A84.1	Electroencephalography Ambulatory
A11.1	Electroencephalography Depth Electrodes Placement
A84.1	Electroencephalography NEC
A11.2	Electroencephalography Surface Electrodes Placement
	Electrofulguration – see Cauterisation
	Electrolysis – see also Epilation
S60.6	Electrolysis Hair
S60.6	Electrolysis NEC
S10.4	Electrolysis Skin Lesion Head
S11.4	Electrolysis Skin Lesion NEC
S10.4	Electrolysis Skin Lesion Neck
A84.2	Electromyography
Y12.3	Electroporation Lesion NOC
A84.-	Electroretinography
V05.3	Elevation Cranium Fracture Depressed
L25.3	Embolectomy Aorta Bifurcation NEC
L26.3	Embolectomy Aorta Bifurcation Transluminal Percutaneous
L38.3	Embolectomy Artery Axillary NEC
L39.2	Embolectomy Artery Axillary Transluminal Percutaneous
L38.3	Embolectomy Artery Brachial NEC
L39.2	Embolectomy Artery Brachial Transluminal Percutaneous
L30.3	Embolectomy Artery Carotid NEC
L34.3	Embolectomy Artery Cerebral NEC
L34.3	Embolectomy Artery Circle Willis NEC
L46.1	Embolectomy Artery Coeliac NEC
L62.2	Embolectomy Artery Femoral NEC
L63.2	Embolectomy Artery Femoral Transluminal Percutaneous
L53.2	Embolectomy Artery Iliac NEC
L54.2	Embolectomy Artery Iliac Transluminal Percutaneous
L46.1	Embolectomy Artery Mesenteric NEC
L70.1	Embolectomy Artery NEC
L62.2	Embolectomy Artery Popliteal NEC
L63.2	Embolectomy Artery Popliteal Transluminal Percutaneous
L12.4	Embolectomy Artery Pulmonary NEC
L13.1	Embolectomy Artery Pulmonary Transluminal Percutaneous
L42.1	Embolectomy Artery Renal NEC
L43.2	Embolectomy Artery Renal Transluminal Percutaneous
L38.3	Embolectomy Artery Subclavian NEC
L39.2	Embolectomy Artery Subclavian Transluminal Percutaneous
L46.1	Embolectomy Artery Suprarenal NEC
L71.2	Embolectomy Artery Transluminal Percutaneous
L38.3	Embolectomy Artery Vertebral NEC
L39.2	Embolectomy Artery Vertebral Transluminal Percutaneous
B25.3	Embolisation Adrenal
L75.-	Embolisation Arteriovenous Abnormality
O05.-	Embolisation Arteriovenous Dural Fistula Transluminal Percutaneous (L)
O02.-	Embolisation Artery Aneurysmal Coil Balloon Assisted Transluminal Percutaneous (L)
O03.-	Embolisation Artery Aneurysmal Coil Stent Assisted Transluminal Percutaneous (L)
O01.-	Embolisation Artery Aneurysmal Coil Transluminal Percutaneous NEC (L)
O04.-	Embolisation Artery Aneurysmal Transluminal Percutaneous NEC (L)

L39.3	Embolisation Artery Axillary NEC
L38.8	Embolisation Artery Axillary Open
L39.3	Embolisation Artery Brachial NEC
L38.8	Embolisation Artery Brachial Open
L35.1	Embolisation Artery Cerebral NEC
L34.4	Embolisation Artery Cerebral Open
L35.1	Embolisation Artery Circle Willis NEC
L34.4	Embolisation Artery Circle Willis Open
L47.2	Embolisation Artery Coeliac NEC
L46.2	Embolisation Artery Coeliac Open
L69.3	Embolisation Artery Collateral Systemic to Pulmonary Transluminal Percutaneous
L63.3	Embolisation Artery Femoral NEC
L62.8	Embolisation Artery Femoral Open
J10.1	Embolisation Artery Hepatic Transluminal Percutaneous
L47.2	Embolisation Artery Mesenteric NEC
L46.2	Embolisation Artery Mesenteric Open
L71.3	Embolisation Artery NEC
E05.3	Embolisation Artery Nose Internal
L70.2	Embolisation Artery Open NEC
L63.3	Embolisation Artery Popliteal NEC
L62.8	Embolisation Artery Popliteal Open
L13.2	Embolisation Artery Pulmonary NEC
L12.5	Embolisation Artery Pulmonary Open
L43.3	Embolisation Artery Renal NEC
L42.2	Embolisation Artery Renal Open
J72.2	Embolisation Artery Splenic
L39.3	Embolisation Artery Subclavian NEC
L38.8	Embolisation Artery Subclavian Open
L47.2	Embolisation Artery Suprarenal NEC
L46.2	Embolisation Artery Suprarenal Open
L71.3	Embolisation Artery Transluminal Percutaneous
L39.3	Embolisation Artery Vertebral NEC
L38.8	Embolisation Artery Vertebral Open
E05.3	Embolisation Nose Internal Artery
J72.2	Embolisation Spleen
N19.2	Embolisation Varicocele
L94.1	Embolisation Vein NEC
J10.2	Embolisation Vein Portal Transluminal Percutaneous
Y70.1	Emergency Operations NOC
	Encirclement – see Cerclage
	Encirclement – see Wiring
L25.-	Endarterectomy Aorta
L37.-	Endarterectomy Artery Axillary
L37.-	Endarterectomy Artery Brachial
L29.-	Endarterectomy Artery Carotid
L45.-	Endarterectomy Artery Coeliac
K47.1	Endarterectomy Artery Coronary
L60.-	Endarterectomy Artery Femoral
L52.-	Endarterectomy Artery Iliac
L45.-	Endarterectomy Artery Mesenteric

L68.-	Endarterectomy Artery NEC
L60.-	Endarterectomy Artery Popliteal
L41.4	Endarterectomy Artery Renal
L37.-	Endarterectomy Artery Subclavian
L45.-	Endarterectomy Artery Suprarenal
L37.-	Endarterectomy Artery Vertebral
Z13.-	Endocrine Gland Neck site
Z14.-	Endocrine Gland site NEC
U29.-	Endocrinology Diagnostic
D26.1	Endolymphatic Sac Operations
	Endoscopic – refer to Index Introduction
	Endoscopic – see Operation site
G80.2	Endoscopy Capsule
G80.2	Endoscopy Wireless Capsule
M36.-	Enlargement Bladder
C29.2	Enlargement Lacrimal Punctum
C05.3	Enlargement Orbit Cavity
K15.1	Enlargement Septum Atrial Defect Closed
K14.1	Enlargement Septum Atrial Defect Open
K14.5	Enlargement Septum Ventricular Defect Open
H19.3	Enterorrhaphy Caecum
H19.3	Enterorrhaphy Colon
G80.-	Enteroscopy NEC
C01.2	Enucleation Eye
C01.2	Enucleation Eyeball
F18.1	Enucleation Jaw Cyst Dental
Y06.3	Enucleation Lesion NOC
A60.1	Enucleation Nerve Peripheral
N15.-	Epididymectomy
N15.-	Epididymis Operations
Z43.3	Epididymis site
N15.7	Epididymovasostomy
Y81.-	Epidural Injection Anaesthetic
A52.-	Epidural Injection Therapeutic
A52.3	Epidural Patch Blood
C22.6	Epilation Eyelash
S60.7	Epilation NEC
V42.2	Epiphysiodesis Joint Spinal Apophyseal
W27.-	Epiphysiodesis NEC
V42.4	Epiphysiodesis Spine Anterior & Posterior
V42.5	Epiphysiodesis Spine Anterior NEC
V42.6	Epiphysiodesis Spine Posterior NEC
W27.2	Epiphysioplasty
R27.1	Episiotomy Delivery
P14.-	Episiotomy Nondelivery
S54.2	Escharotomy Skin Burnt Head
S55.2	Escharotomy Skin Burnt NEC
S54.2	Escharotomy Skin Burnt Neck
S56.2	Escharotomy Skin Head NEC
S57.2	Escharotomy Skin NEC

S56.2	Escharotomy Skin Neck NEC
S54.2	Escharotomy Subcutaneous Tissue Burnt Head
S55.2	Escharotomy Subcutaneous Tissue Burnt NEC
S54.2	Escharotomy Subcutaneous Tissue Burnt Neck
S56.2	Escharotomy Subcutaneous Tissue Head NEC
S57.2	Escharotomy Subcutaneous Tissue NEC
S56.2	Escharotomy Subcutaneous Tissue Neck NEC
E85.2	Establishing Pressure Airway Continuous Positive
E85.2	Establishing Pressure Chest-wall Continuous Negative
E14.-	Ethmoid Operations
E14.-	Ethmoid Sinus Operations
Z23.3	Ethmoid Sinus site
E14.-	Ethmoidectomy NEC
D22.-	Eustachian Canal Operations
Z21.3	Eustachian Canal site
	Evacuation – see also Aspiration
	Evacuation – see also Drainage
Y44.1	Evacuation Contents NOC
A40.1	Evacuation Extradural Haematoma
H53.1	Evacuation Haemorrhoid Thrombosed
H53.1	Evacuation Perianal Haematoma
H44.3	Evacuation Rectum Faeces Impacted Manual
T96.4	Evacuation Soft Tissue Seroma
A41.1	Evacuation Subdural Haematoma
Q11.-	Evacuation Uterus Contents NEC
Q11.-	Evacuation Uterus Products Conception
P27.1	Evacuation Vagina Haematoma
P09.3	Evacuation Vulva Haematoma
X50.5	Evaluation Cardioverter Defibrillator
X50.5	Evaluation Cardioverter Defibrillator Subcutaneous Induction Ventricular Fibrillation
X50.5	Evaluation Cardioverter Defibrillator Transvenous Induction Ventricular Fibrillation
C87.-	Evaluation Retina
C87.1	Evaluation Retina Electrodiagnostic
C87.2	Evaluation Retina Indocyanine Angiography
C87.5	Evaluation Retina Scanning Laser Ophthalmoscopy
C87.3	Evaluation Retina Tomography
C87.4	Evaluation Retina Ultrasound
N11.3	Eversion Hydrocele Sac
B35.6	Eversion Nipple
C01.3	Evisceration Eye
C01.3	Evisceration Eyeball Contents
A84.4	Evoked Potential Recording
Y41.-	Examination Anaesthetic NOC
J43.-	Examination Bile Duct & Pancreatic Duct Endoscopic Retrograde
J44.-	Examination Bile Duct Endoscopic Retrograde
J53.-	Examination Bile Duct Endoscopic Ultrasonic
J51.-	Examination Bile Duct Laparoscopic Ultrasound
J50.-	Examination Bile Duct Percutaneous
J50.6	Examination Bile Duct Percutaneous Transjejunal NEC
M45.-	Examination Bladder Endoscopic

H25.-	Examination Bowel Lower Sigmoidoscope Fibreoptic
A18.-	Examination Brain Ventricle Endoscopic Diagnostic
E49.-	Examination Bronchus Endoscopic NEC
E51.-	Examination Bronchus Endoscopic Rigid
H22.-	Examination Caecum Endoscopic Fibreoptic
H22.-	Examination Caecum Endoscopic NEC
U17.6	Examination Capsule Patency
E49.-	Examination Carina Endoscopic NEC
E51.-	Examination Carina Endoscopic Rigid
Q55.-	Examination Cervix Uteri NEC
H22.-	Examination Colon Endoscopic Fibreoptic NEC
H22.-	Examination Colon Endoscopic NEC
H25.-	Examination Colon Sigmoid Endoscopic NEC
H25.-	Examination Colon Sigmoid Sigmoidoscope Fibreoptic
H28.-	Examination Colon Sigmoid Sigmoidoscope Rigid
H25.-	Examination Colon Sigmoidoscope Fibreoptic
H68.2	Examination Colonic Pouch Colonoscope
H69.2	Examination Colonic Pouch Sigmoidoscope Flexible
H70.2	Examination Colonic Pouch Sigmoidoscope Rigid
G55.-	Examination Duodenum Endoscopic NEC
D28.2	Examination Ear Anaesthetic
C86.6	Examination Eye Anaesthetic
Q39.-	Examination Fallopian Tube Endoscopic
R02.-	Examination Fetus Endoscopic
R05.-	Examination Fetus Percutaneous
J09.-	Examination Gall Bladder Endoscopic
G45.-	Examination Gastrointestinal Tract Upper Endoscopic Fibreoptic
G45.-	Examination Gastrointestinal Tract Upper Endoscopic NEC
G45.2	Examination Gastrointestinal Tract Upper Ultrasound Endoscopic
Q55.-	Examination Genital Tract Female Anaesthetic
Q55.-	Examination Genital Tract Female NEC
Q55.5	Examination Genital Tract Female Ultrasound Transvaginal
Q55.-	Examination Gynaecological Anaesthetic
H68.4	Examination Ileoanal Pouch Colonoscope
H69.4	Examination Ileoanal Pouch Sigmoidoscope Flexible
H70.4	Examination Ileoanal Pouch Sigmoidoscope Rigid
G80.-	Examination Ileum Endoscopic
G80.3	Examination Ileum Endoscopic Balloon Diagnostic
G80.-	Examination Intestine Small Endoscopic NEC
G65.-	Examination Jejunum Endoscopic
W88.-	Examination Joint Endoscopic NEC
W87.-	Examination Joint Knee Endoscopic
W92.-	Examination Joint NEC
M11.-	Examination Kidney Endoscopic
M11.3	Examination Kidney Endoscopic Retrograde NEC
M17.5	Examination Kidney Post-transplantation Live Donor
M17.4	Examination Kidney Post-transplantation Recipient
E36.-	Examination Larynx Endoscopic
E37.-	Examination Larynx Microendoscopic Diagnostic
J09.-	Examination Liver Endoscopic NEC

J17.-	Examination Liver Endoscopic Ultrasonic
J09.-	Examination Liver Laparoscopic Ultrasonic
E49.-	Examination Lung Endoscopic NEC
E51.-	Examination Lung Endoscopic Rigid
E63.-	Examination Mediastinum Endoscopic
E63.3	Examination Mediastinum Ultrasound Endo-oesophageal
E63.2	Examination Mediastinum Ultrasound Endobronchial
F43.-	Examination Mouth Other
E65.-	Examination Nasal Cavity Endoscopic
E27.6	Examination Nasopharynx Anaesthetic
E25.-	Examination Nasopharynx Endoscopic
Y41.-	Examination NOC
G16.-	Examination Oesophagus Endoscopic Fibreoptic NEC
G16.-	Examination Oesophagus Endoscopic NEC
G16.2	Examination Oesophagus Ultrasound Endoscopic Fibreoptic
Q50.-	Examination Ovary Endoscopic
J74.-	Examination Pancreas Endoscopic Ultrasonic
J73.-	Examination Pancreas Laparoscopic Ultrasonic
J63.-	Examination Pancreas Open
J43.-	Examination Pancreatic Duct & Bile Duct Endoscopic Retrograde
J45.-	Examination Pancreatic Duct Endoscopic Retrograde
T43.-	Examination Peritoneal Cavity Endoscopic
T43.-	Examination Peritoneal Cavity Endoscopic Ultrasonic
T43.-	Examination Peritoneum Endoscopic
E27.6	Examination Pharynx Anaesthetic
E25.-	Examination Pharynx Endoscopic
R05.-	Examination Placenta Percutaneous
T11.-	Examination Pleura Endoscopic
T11.-	Examination Pleural Cavity Endoscopic
H68.-	Examination Pouch Colonoscope
H69.-	Examination Pouch Sigmoidoscope Flexible
H70.-	Examination Pouch Sigmoidoscope Rigid
G45.-	Examination Pylorus Endoscopic Fibreoptic
G45.-	Examination Pylorus Endoscopic NEC
H44.4	Examination Rectum Anaesthetic
H25.-	Examination Rectum Endoscopic NEC
H25.-	Examination Rectum Sigmoidoscope Fibreoptic
H28.-	Examination Rectum Sigmoidoscope Rigid
E49.-	Examination Respiratory Tract Lower Endoscopic NEC
E51.-	Examination Respiratory Tract Lower Endoscopic Rigid
G45.-	Examination Stomach Endoscopic Fibreoptic
G45.-	Examination Stomach Endoscopic NEC
G19.-	Examination Stomach Gastroscope Rigid
E49.-	Examination Trachea Endoscopic NEC
E51.-	Examination Trachea Endoscopic Rigid
	Examination Ultrasound Endoscopic – see Examination site
	Examination Under Anaesthetic – see Examination site
M30.5	Examination Ureter & Biopsy Endoscopic NEC
M30.6	Examination Ureter & Biopsy Ureteroscope Rigid
M30.-	Examination Ureter Endoscopic

M77.-	Examination Urethra Endoscopic
M85.-	Examination Urinary Diversion Endoscopic
Q18.-	Examination Uterus Endoscopic
Q55.-	Examination Uterus NEC
Q55.-	Examination Vagina NEC
Q55.5	Examination Vagina Ultrasound
U11.-	Examination Vascular Ultrasound
	Exchange Fluid – see Transfusion
	Excision – see also Extirpation
	Excision – see also Resection
T31.-	Excision Abdominal Wall Anterior Lesion
T31.-	Excision Abdominal Wall Lesion NEC
T39.1	Excision Abdominal Wall Posterior Lesion
E20.1	Excision Adenoid
B22.-	Excision Adrenal
B25.1	Excision Adrenal Lesion
B23.1	Excision Adrenal Tissue Aberrant Lesion
J36.1	Excision Ampulla Vater
J27.1	Excision Ampulla Vater & Replantation Bile Duct Common
X12.2	Excision Amputation Stump Lesion
H56.4	Excision Anal Fissure
	Excision Aneurysm – see Operation site Aneurysmal
H47.-	Excision Anus
H48.-	Excision Anus Lesion
H01.-	Excision Appendix Emergency
H02.-	Excision Appendix NEC
S03.3	Excision Arm Fat Redundant
L75.1	Excision Arteriovenous Malformation Congenital
L33.1	Excision Artery Cerebral Aneurysmal
L33.1	Excision Artery Circle Willis Aneurysmal
L67.-	Excision Artery NEC
	Excision Arthroplasty – see Arthroplasty site
K22.1	Excision Atrium Lesion
D08.1	Excision Auditory Canal External Lesion
V54.1	Excision Axis Odontoid Process Transoral
P03.-	Excision Bartholin Gland
J27.-	Excision Bile Duct
J27.5	Excision Bile Duct Extrahepatic
J28.1	Excision Bile Duct Lesion
J27.5	Excision Biliary Tree Extrahepatic
	Excision Biopsy Lesion – see Excision Lesion
M41.1	Excision Bladder Lesion Open
M35.-	Excision Bladder Partial
M34.-	Excision Bladder Total
W08.3	Excision Bone Calcium Deposit
W07.1	Excision Bone Cross Union
W07.-	Excision Bone Ectopic
W08.3	Excision Bone Excrescence
V07.-	Excision Bone Face
W06.5	Excision Bone Foot Total NEC

W08.4	Excision Bone Fragment
W21.2	Excision Bone Fragment Intra-articular Fracture Primary
W09.-	Excision Bone Lesion
W03.1	Excision Bone Metatarsal Lesser Multiple Head
W08.-	Excision Bone NEC
W08.2	Excision Bone Overgrowth
W06.7	Excision Bone Pelvis Total
W06.4	Excision Bone Sesamoid Total NEC
W06.-	Excision Bone Total
W08.1	Excision Bone Tuberosity
A38.-	Excision Brain Meninges Lesion
A02.6	Excision Brain Stem Tissue Lesion
A07.4	Excision Brain Tissue Abscess
A02.-	Excision Brain Tissue Lesion
A06.-	Excision Brain Tissue Lesion Other
A01.-	Excision Brain Tissue Major
T94.1	Excision Branchial Cyst
B28.6	Excision Breast Accessory Tissue
B28.3	Excision Breast Lesion NEC
B28.7	Excision Breast Lesion Wire Guided
B28.-	Excision Breast NEC
B28.-	Excision Breast Partial
B28.1	Excision Breast Quadrant
B27.-	Excision Breast Total
B28.-	Excision Breast Wedge
B28.-	Excision Breast Wide
B28.-	Excision Breast Wire Guided
E46.-	Excision Bronchus Lesion
E46.-	Excision Bronchus Partial
W79.2	Excision Bunion NEC
W79.2	Excision Bunionette
T62.-	Excision Bursa
H06.-	Excision Caecum Extended
H12.-	Excision Caecum Lesion
H07.-	Excision Caecum NEC
C11.1	Excision Canthus Lesion
E44.-	Excision Carina
W83.6	Excision Cartilage Articular Endoscopic NEC
W82.-	Excision Cartilage Semilunar Endoscopic
W70.-	Excision Cartilage Semilunar NEC
Q01.-	Excision Cervix Uteri
T01.3	Excision Chest Wall Lesion
T01.-	Excision Chest Wall Partial
C84.2	Excision Choroid Lesion
C66.-	Excision Ciliary Body
W06.6	Excision Coccyx Total
H29.-	Excision Colon & Rectum Subtotal
H04.-	Excision Colon & Rectum Total
H09.-	Excision Colon Left
H20.6	Excision Colon Lesion Endoscopic Fibreoptic NEC

H12.-	Excision Colon Lesion NEC
H11.-	Excision Colon NEC
H29.-	Excision Colon Partial
H06.-	Excision Colon Right Extended
H07.-	Excision Colon Right NEC
H10.-	Excision Colon Sigmoid NEC
H33.-	Excision Colon Sigmoid Part & Rectum
H29.-	Excision Colon Subtotal
H05.-	Excision Colon Total NEC
H08.-	Excision Colon Transverse NEC
C39.1	Excision Conjunctiva Lesion
C45.2	Excision Cornea Lesion NEC
V05.1	Excision Cranium Lesion
T96.1	Excision Cystic Hygroma
T17.1	Excision Diaphragm Lesion
V58.-	Excision Disc Intervertebral Automated Mechanical Percutaneous NEC
V58.-	Excision Disc Intervertebral Automated Mechanical Percutaneous Primary
V59.-	Excision Disc Intervertebral Automated Mechanical Percutaneous Revisional
V29.-	Excision Disc Intervertebral Cervical NEC
V30.-	Excision Disc Intervertebral Cervical Revisional
V58.3	Excision Disc Intervertebral Lumbar Automated Mechanical Percutaneous NEC
V59.3	Excision Disc Intervertebral Lumbar Automated Mechanical Percutaneous Revisional
V33.-	Excision Disc Intervertebral Lumbar NEC
V34.-	Excision Disc Intervertebral Lumbar Revisional
V35.-	Excision Disc Intervertebral NEC
V35.2	Excision Disc Intervertebral Revisional NEC
V31.-	Excision Disc Intervertebral Thoracic NEC
V32.-	Excision Disc Intervertebral Thoracic Revisional
G70.1	Excision Diverticulum Meckel's
G49.-	Excision Duodenum
G50.1	Excision Duodenum Lesion NEC
D01.-	Excision Ear External
D02.1	Excision Ear External Lesion
D02.1	Excision Ear External Skin Lesion
D19.1	Excision Ear Middle Lesion
A06.-	Excision Encephalocele
N15.3	Excision Epididymis Hydatid Morgagni
N15.3	Excision Epididymis Lesion
C01.-	Excision Eye
C37.1	Excision Eye Muscle Lesion
C10.1	Excision Eyebrow Lesion
C10.1	Excision Eyebrow Skin Lesion
C12.1	Excision Eyelid Lesion NEC
C12.6	Excision Eyelid Lesion Wedge
C12.1	Excision Eyelid Skin Lesion
C13.-	Excision Eyelid Skin Redundant
Q25.-	Excision Fallopian Tube Partial
A38.5	Excision Falx Cerebri Lesion
T51.-	Excision Fascia Abdomen
T53.1	Excision Fascia Lesion

T52.-	Excision Fascia NEC
T56.-	Excision Fascia Other NEC
T51.2	Excision Fascia Pelvis
X23.3	Excision Fibula Anlage
Q32.1	Excision Fimbria
Q32.3	Excision Fimbria Hydatid Morgagni
Y05.3	Excision Fistula NOC
J23.1	Excision Gall Bladder Lesion NEC
J18.-	Excision Gall Bladder NEC
T59.-	Excision Ganglion
F20.-	Excision Gingiva
F20.2	Excision Gingiva Lesion
X16.3	Excision Gonad Abdomen
X16.5	Excision Gonad Inguinal Canal
X16.6	Excision Gonad NEC
X16.4	Excision Gonad Pelvis
X16.3	Excision Gonad Streak from Abdomen
X16.5	Excision Gonad Streak from Inguinal Canal
X16.4	Excision Gonad Streak from Pelvis
X16.6	Excision Gonad Streak NEC
H51.-	Excision Haemorrhoid
K52.-	Excision Heart Rhythmogenic Focus
K36.-	Excision Heart Valve NEC
K34.4	Excision Heart Valve Vegetations
K23.1	Excision Heart Ventricle Lesion
K23.1	Excision Heart Wall Lesion NEC
T19.-	Excision Hernial Sac Inguinal Simple
Q32.3	Excision Hydatid Morgagni Female
N11.1	Excision Hydrocele Sac
P15.2	Excision Hymenal Tag
H66.1	Excision Ileoanal Pouch
G69.-	Excision Ileum
G79.1	Excision Ileum Lesion Endoscopic
G70.2	Excision Ileum Lesion NEC
V07.4	Excision Infratemporal Fossa Lesion
G79.1	Excision Intestine Small Lesion Endoscopic NEC
G70.2	Excision Intestine Small Lesion NEC
G69.-	Excision Intestine Small NEC
C59.-	Excision Iris
C64.2	Excision Iris Lesion
C64.1	Excision Iris Prolapsed
J58.1	Excision Islet Langerhans Lesion
F18.-	Excision Jaw Lesion Dental
V14.-	Excision Jaw NEC
G58.-	Excision Jejunum
G59.1	Excision Jejunum Lesion
G64.1	Excision Jejunum Lesion Endoscopic
	Excision Joint – see Decompression
O19.2	Excision Joint Knee Infrapatellar Fat Pad Endoscopic (W)
W81.1	Excision Joint Lesion NEC

W71.2	Excision Joint Osteophyte
M04.2	Excision Kidney Lesion Open NEC
M02.-	Excision Kidney NEC
M03.-	Excision Kidney Partial
M02.7	Excision Kidney Transplanted NEC
M02.6	Excision Kidney Transplanted Rejected
P05.5	Excision Labial Tissue Excess
C24.1	Excision Lacrimal Gland
C26.1	Excision Lacrimal Sac
E29.-	Excision Larynx
E35.2	Excision Larynx Lesion Endoscopic NEC
E30.-	Excision Larynx Lesion Open
Y08.-	Excision Laser NOC
L87.5	Excision Leg Vein Varicose Local
	Excision Lesion – see also Excision site
	Excision Lesion – see also Excision site Partial
	Excision Lesion – see also Resection site
Y06.-	Excision Lesion NOC
W76.-	Excision Ligament
F02.1	Excision Lip Lesion
F05.1	Excision Lip Mucosa Excess
F02.1	Excision Lip Mucosa Lesion
F01.-	Excision Lip Partial
F02.1	Excision Lip Skin Lesion
F01.-	Excision Lip Skin Partial
F01.1	Excision Lip Vermilion Border & Advancement Mucosa
J03.1	Excision Liver Lesion
J03.5	Excision Liver Lesion Multiple
J02.-	Excision Liver Partial
E55.2	Excision Lung Lesion NEC
E54.-	Excision Lung NEC
T87.-	Excision Lymph Node NEC
T92.1	Excision Lymphocele
T92.-	Excision Lymphoedematous Tissue
B34.-	Excision Mammary Duct
V14.-	Excision Mandible
D10.-	Excision Mastoid
V06.-	Excision Maxilla
E13.2	Excision Maxillary Antrum Lesion
E62.1	Excision Mediastinum Lesion Endoscopic
E61.1	Excision Mediastinum Lesion Open
A43.1	Excision Meninges Skull Base Lesion
A43.2	Excision Meninges Skull Clivus Lesion
T38.1	Excision Mesentery Colon Lesion
T37.1	Excision Mesentery Intestine Small Lesion
W03.-	Excision Metatarsal Head Multiple
F38.-	Excision Mouth Lesion NEC
F42.3	Excision Mouth Mucosa Excess NEC
X16.1	Excision Mullerian Duct Remnant
X16.2	Excision Mullerian Duct Remnant Lesion

T77.-	Excision Muscle
C37.1	Excision Muscle Eye Lesion
S68.-	Excision Nail
S64.1	Excision Nail Bed
E17.2	Excision Nasal Sinus Lesion NEC
E17.1	Excision Nasal Sinus NEC
E19.-	Excision Nasopharynx
E24.1	Excision Nasopharynx Lesion Endoscopic
E23.1	Excision Nasopharynx Lesion Open
	Excision Nerve – see also Avulsion Nerve
	Excision Nerve – see also Denervation
	Excision Nerve – see also Sacrifice Nerve
	Excision Nerve – see also Transection Nerve
A29.-	Excision Nerve Cranial Lesion
A59.-	Excision Nerve Peripheral
A61.1	Excision Nerve Peripheral Lesion
A59.-	Excision Nerve Peripheral Sacrifice
A57.1	Excision Nerve Root Spinal Lesion
A75.-	Excision Nerve Sympathetic
A27.-	Excision Nerve Vagus (x) NEC
E13.7	Excision Nerve Vidian NEC
B35.-	Excision Nipple
B35.-	Excision Nipple Skin
Y05.-	Excision NOC
E01.-	Excision Nose
E09.1	Excision Nose External Lesion
E09.1	Excision Nose External Skin Lesion
E08.2	Excision Nose Internal Lesion NEC
E03.2	Excision Nose Septum Lesion
E03.1	Excision Nose Septum Submucous
E04.-	Excision Nose Turbinate
G01.-	Excision Oesophagus & Stomach
G07.-	Excision Oesophagus Fistula
G04.1	Excision Oesophagus Lesion
G03.-	Excision Oesophagus NEC
G02.-	Excision Oesophagus Total
T36.2	Excision Omentum Lesion
C13.-	Excision Orbit Fat
C02.1	Excision Orbit Lesion
Y06.7	Excision Organ Lesion Radiofrequency
Y06.6	Excision Organ Lesion Vacuum
X53.-	Excision Organ Unspecified
W08.7	Excision Ossicle Accessory
W71.2	Excision Osteophyte Intra-articular
Q43.2	Excision Ovary Lesion
Q49.1	Excision Ovary Lesion Endoscopic
Q43.-	Excision Ovary Partial
Q43.1	Excision Ovary Wedge
X16.3	Excision Ovotestis from Abdomen
X16.5	Excision Ovotestis from Inguinal Canal

X16.4	Excision Ovotestis from Pelvis
X16.6	Excision Ovotestis NEC
F28.1	Excision Palate Lesion
J56.-	Excision Pancreas Head
J58.2	Excision Pancreas Lesion NEC
J57.-	Excision Pancreas Partial NEC
J57.-	Excision Pancreas Tail
J55.-	Excision Pancreas Total
J55.3	Excision Pancreas Transplanted
J36.1	Excision Papilla Vater
B14.-	Excision Parathyroid
W06.3	Excision Patella Total
N27.1	Excision Penis Lesion
N27.1	Excision Penis Skin Lesion
H48.-	Excision Perianal Region Lesion
K67.-	Excision Pericardium
K67.1	Excision Pericardium Lesion
P11.1	Excision Perineum Female Lesion
P11.1	Excision Perineum Skin Female Lesion
P13.7	Excision Perineum Skin Sweat Gland Bearing Female
N24.1	Excision Perineum Skin Sweat Gland Bearing Male
T33.1	Excision Peritoneum Lesion Open
T39.1	Excision Peritoneum Posterior Lesion
N24.3	Excision Periurethral Tissue Male NEC
Q07.-	Excision Periuterine Tissue & Hysterectomy Abdominal NEC
Q08.-	Excision Periuterine Tissue & Hysterectomy Vaginal NEC
E19.-	Excision Pharynx
E24.2	Excision Pharynx Lesion Endoscopic
E23.1	Excision Pharynx Lesion Open
H59.-	Excision Pilonidal Abscess
H59.-	Excision Pilonidal Cyst
H59.-	Excision Pilonidal Sinus
B06.1	Excision Pineal
B01.-	Excision Pituitary
B04.1	Excision Pituitary Lesion
T10.1	Excision Pleura Lesion Endoscopic
T07.-	Excision Pleura Open
D01.3	Excision Preauricular Abnormality
M61.1	Excision Prostate & Capsule Total
M62.1	Excision Prostate Lesion Open
M61.-	Excision Prostate Open
X20.1	Excision Radius Anlage
H33.-	Excision Rectum
H33.-	Excision Rectum & Colon Sigmoid Part
H29.-	Excision Rectum & Colon Subtotal
H04.-	Excision Rectum & Colon Total
H33.1	Excision Rectum Abdominoperineal & Colostomy End
H34.1	Excision Rectum Lesion Open
H41.2	Excision Rectum Lesion Peranal
H40.2	Excision Rectum Lesion Trans-sphincteric

H40.1	Excision Rectum Mucosa Trans-sphincteric
H42.5	Excision Rectum Prolapse Mucosal NEC
C84.2	Excision Retina Lesion
T08.1	Excision Rib & Drainage Pleural Cavity Open
V42.1	Excision Rib Hump
W06.-	Excision Rib Total
F44.-	Excision Salivary Gland
F45.-	Excision Salivary Gland Lesion
	Excision Scar – see Refashioning Scar
Y06.4	Excision Scar Tissue NOC
C52.-	Excision Sclera
C53.2	Excision Sclera Lesion NEC
N01.-	Excision Scrotum
N01.-	Excision Scrotum Skin
N22.1	Excision Seminal Vesicle
Y05.3	Excision Sinus Track NOC
S02.-	Excision Skin Abdominal Wall Plastic
S54.2	Excision Skin Burnt Head
S55.2	Excision Skin Burnt NEC
S54.2	Excision Skin Burnt Neck
S56.1	Excision Skin Devitalised Head NEC
S57.1	Excision Skin Devitalised NEC
S56.1	Excision Skin Devitalised Neck NEC
S01.-	Excision Skin Head Plastic
S05.-	Excision Skin Lesion Microscopically Controlled
S06.-	Excision Skin Lesion NEC
S04.-	Excision Skin NEC
S01.-	Excision Skin Neck Plastic
S03.-	Excision Skin Plastic NEC
S03.3	Excision Skin Redundant Arm
S04.-	Excision Skin Sweat Gland Bearing
T96.2	Excision Soft Tissue Lesion NEC
N20.1	Excision Spermatic Cord Hydatid Morgagni
N20.1	Excision Spermatic Cord Lesion
E15.4	Excision Sphenoid Sinus Lesion
J36.1	Excision Sphincter Oddi
A44.4	Excision Spinal Cord Extradural Lesion
A44.5	Excision Spinal Cord Intradural Extramedullary Lesion
A44.3	Excision Spinal Cord Intradural Intramedullary Lesion
A44.2	Excision Spinal Cord Lesion NEC
A51.1	Excision Spinal Cord Meninges Lesion
A44.-	Excision Spinal Cord Partial
V43.-	Excision Spine Lesion
J69.3	Excision Spleen Accessory
J70.-	Excision Spleen NEC
J69.-	Excision Spleen Total
J69.1	Excision Spleen Total & Replantation Spleen Fragments
G01.-	Excision Stomach & Oesophagus
G29.-	Excision Stomach Lesion Open
G28.-	Excision Stomach Partial

G28.5	Excision Stomach Partial Sleeve
G28.4	Excision Stomach Partial Sleeve & Duodenal Switch
G28.-	Excision Stomach Sleeve
G27.-	Excision Stomach Total
S02.-	Excision Subcutaneous Tissue Abdominal Wall Plastic
S54.2	Excision Subcutaneous Tissue Burnt Head
S55.2	Excision Subcutaneous Tissue Burnt NEC
S54.2	Excision Subcutaneous Tissue Burnt Neck
S56.1	Excision Subcutaneous Tissue Devitalised Head NEC
S57.1	Excision Subcutaneous Tissue Devitalised NEC
S56.1	Excision Subcutaneous Tissue Devitalised Neck NEC
S01.-	Excision Subcutaneous Tissue Head Plastic
S05.-	Excision Subcutaneous Tissue Lesion Microscopically Controlled
S06.-	Excision Subcutaneous Tissue Lesion NEC
S01.-	Excision Subcutaneous Tissue Neck Plastic
S03.-	Excision Subcutaneous Tissue Plastic NEC
K37.5	Excision Supramitral Ring
W84.6	Excision Synovial Plica Endoscopic
	Excision Tattoo – see Excision Skin Lesion
T65.2	Excision Tendon Lesion
T65.-	Excision Tendon NEC
T65.1	Excision Tendon Sacrifice
T71.-	Excision Tendon Sheath
A38.6	Excision Tentorium Cerebelli Lesion
N06.4	Excision Testicular Appendage
N06.2	Excision Testis Aberrant
N05.-	Excision Testis Bilateral
X16.3	Excision Testis from Abdomen Female
X16.6	Excision Testis from Female NEC
X16.5	Excision Testis from Inguinal Canal Female
X16.4	Excision Testis from Pelvis Female
N07.1	Excision Testis Hydatid Morgagni
N06.6	Excision Testis Inguinal & Excision Cord Spermatic NEC
N05.3	Excision Testis Inguinal Bilateral
N05.3	Excision Testis Inguinal Bilateral & Excision Cord Spermatic
N06.6	Excision Testis Inguinal NEC
N07.1	Excision Testis Lesion
N06.-	Excision Testis NEC
B18.-	Excision Thymus
B10.1	Excision Thyroglossal Cyst
B10.2	Excision Thyroglossal Tract
B08.-	Excision Thyroid
B12.1	Excision Thyroid Lesion
B09.2	Excision Thyroid Tissue Sublingual
B09.1	Excision Thyroid Tissue Substernal
X23.4	Excision Tibia Anlage
F22.-	Excision Tongue
F26.2	Excision Tongue Frenulum
F23.1	Excision Tongue Lesion
F34.-	Excision Tonsil

F36.6	Excision Tonsil Lesion
E39.1	Excision Trachea Lesion NEC
E39.-	Excision Trachea Partial
A02.7	Excision Transcranial Dermoid Cyst
Q01.4	Excision Transformation Zone Large Loop
V05.6	Excision Transpetrous Lesion Jugular Foramen
X20.2	Excision Ulna Anlage
T29.1	Excision Umbilicus
T29.5	Excision Umbilicus Fistula
T29.3	Excision Umbilicus Lesion
T29.5	Excision Umbilicus Sinus
T29.2	Excision Urachus
M18.-	Excision Ureter
M18.4	Excision Ureter Duplex
M25.2	Excision Ureter Lesion Open
M32.1	Excision Ureteric Orifice Lesion Endoscopic
M25.1	Excision Ureterocele
M72.-	Excision Urethra
M76.1	Excision Urethra Lesion Endoscopic
M81.1	Excision Urethra Meatus Lesion
X16.1	Excision Uterine Horn
Q07.-	Excision Uterus Abdominal
Q07.6	Excision Uterus Accessory
Q22.-	Excision Uterus Adnexa Bilateral
Q24.-	Excision Uterus Adnexa NEC
Q23.-	Excision Uterus Adnexa Unilateral
Q09.3	Excision Uterus Lesion NEC
Q16.1	Excision Uterus Lesion Vaginal
Q52.1	Excision Uterus Ligament Broad Lesion
Q07.4	Excision Uterus NEC
X16.1	Excision Uterus Rudimentary
Q08.-	Excision Uterus Vaginal
P17.-	Excision Vagina
P19.-	Excision Vagina Band
P20.1	Excision Vagina Lesion
P19.-	Excision Vagina Septum
N17.-	Excision Vas Deferens
L93.6	Excision Vein Lesion NEC
L93.1	Excision Vein NEC
L79.7	Excision Vena Cava Lesion
V43.-	Excision Vertebra Lesion
C79.-	Excision Vitreous Body
C79.1	Excision Vitreous Body Anterior Approach
C79.2	Excision Vitreous Body NEC
C79.2	Excision Vitreous Body Pars Plana Approach
P05.-	Excision Vulva
P05.-	Excision Vulva Lesion
P05.-	Excision Vulva Skin
P06.-	Excision Vulva Skin Lesion
K22.3	Exclusion Atrial Appendage Left NEC

K62.5	Exclusion Atrial Appendage Left Transluminal Percutaneous
G78.5	Exclusion Ileum Segment
G78.5	Exclusion Intestine Small Segment NEC
D10.-	Exenteration Mastoid Air Cells
C01.1	Exenteration Orbit
X14.-	Exenteration Pelvis
X14.1	Exenteration Pelvis NEC
S49.-	Expander Skin Attention
S48.-	Expander Skin Insertion
V02.2	Expansion Calvarium
C55.4	Expansion Sclera
E89.2	Expectoration Respiratory Tract Sputum Induced
C54.6	Explant Sclera Removal
	Exploration – see also Examination
	Exploration – see also Operation site
	Exploration – see also Re-exploration
B25.4	Exploration Adrenal
B23.2	Exploration Adrenal Tissue Aberrant
K48.4	Exploration Artery Coronary
J33.-	Exploration Bile Duct NEC
M41.5	Exploration Bladder
A07.3	Exploration Brain Tissue
B33.3	Exploration Breast
T62.6	Exploration Bursa
C43.5	Exploration Conjunctiva
C51.3	Exploration Cornea
D15.3	Exploration Ear Middle
C22.5	Exploration Eyelid
Q34.4	Exploration Fallopian Tube
Y31.1	Exploration Fistula NOC
J23.3	Exploration Gall Bladder
T30.4	Exploration Groin & Opening Abdomen
T31.7	Exploration Groin NEC
K53.2	Exploration Heart NEC
W81.5	Exploration Joint NEC
M08.-	Exploration Kidney
J07.3	Exploration Liver
B34.5	Exploration Mammary Duct
D12.4	Exploration Mastoid
E61.5	Exploration Mediastinum
T83.4	Exploration Muscle
A34.-	Exploration Nerve Cranial
A73.4	Exploration Nerve Peripheral
Y31.-	Exploration NOC
C06.5	Exploration Orbit
B16.3	Exploration Parathyroid
K71.4	Exploration Pericardium
B04.4	Exploration Pituitary
M83.2	Exploration Retropubic Space
	Exploration Scar – see Exploration Skin

N03.4	Exploration Scrotum
Y31.1	Exploration Sinus Track NOC
S54.-	Exploration Skin Burnt Head
S55.-	Exploration Skin Burnt NEC
S54.-	Exploration Skin Burnt Neck
S56.-	Exploration Skin Head NEC
S57.-	Exploration Skin NEC
S56.-	Exploration Skin Neck NEC
V49.-	Exploration Spine
S54.-	Exploration Subcutaneous Tissue Burnt Head
S55.-	Exploration Subcutaneous Tissue Burnt NEC
S54.-	Exploration Subcutaneous Tissue Burnt Neck
S56.-	Exploration Subcutaneous Tissue Head NEC
S57.-	Exploration Subcutaneous Tissue NEC
S56.-	Exploration Subcutaneous Tissue Neck NEC
T74.3	Exploration Tendon NEC
T72.4	Exploration Tendon Sheath
N13.5	Exploration Testis
B20.2	Exploration Thymus
B12.4	Exploration Thyroid
M25.5	Exploration Ureter Open
R30.-	Exploration Uterus Delivered
Q20.5	Exploration Uterus NEC
P27.-	Exploration Vagina
F14.5	Exposure Tooth Surgical
R30.2	Expression Placenta
	Exteriorisation – see also Opening
H03.3	Exteriorisation Appendix
H09.5	Exteriorisation Bowel & Excision Colon Left
H11.5	Exteriorisation Bowel & Excision Colon NEC
H10.5	Exteriorisation Bowel & Excision Colon Sigmoid NEC
H08.5	Exteriorisation Bowel & Excision Colon Transverse NEC
H33.-	Exteriorisation Bowel & Excision Rectum
H14.-	Exteriorisation Caecum
H32.-	Exteriorisation Colon
H15.-	Exteriorisation Colon Other NEC
Y16.1	Exteriorisation NOC
G08.1	Exteriorisation Oesophagus Pouch
E42.-	Exteriorisation Trachea
	Extirpation – see also Avulsion
	Extirpation – see also Destruction
	Extirpation – see also Excision
D08.1	Extirpation Auditory Canal External Lesion
J28.-	Extirpation Bile Duct Lesion
M42.-	Extirpation Bladder Lesion Endoscopic
M41.1	Extirpation Bladder Lesion Open
W09.-	Extirpation Bone Lesion
H23.-	Extirpation Bowel Lower Lesion Sigmoidoscope Fibreoptic
A38.-	Extirpation Brain Meninges Lesion
A17.1	Extirpation Brain Ventricle Lesion Endoscopic

E46.-	Extirpation Bronchus Partial
H20.-	Extirpation Caecum Lesion Endoscopic Fibreoptic
H20.-	Extirpation Caecum Lesion Endoscopic NEC
H12.-	Extirpation Caecum Lesion NEC
C66.-	Extirpation Ciliary Body
H20.-	Extirpation Colon Lesion Endoscopic Fibreoptic
H20.-	Extirpation Colon Lesion Endoscopic NEC
H12.-	Extirpation Colon Lesion NEC
H23.-	Extirpation Colon Lesion Sigmoidoscope Fibreoptic
H23.-	Extirpation Colon Sigmoid Lesion Endoscopic NEC
H23.-	Extirpation Colon Sigmoid Lesion Sigmoidoscope Fibreoptic
H26.-	Extirpation Colon Sigmoid Lesion Sigmoidoscope Rigid
C39.-	Extirpation Conjunctiva Lesion
C45.-	Extirpation Cornea Lesion
V05.1	Extirpation Cranium Lesion
G54.1	Extirpation Duodenum Lesion Endoscopic NEC
G50.-	Extirpation Duodenum Lesion Open
G43.-	Extirpation Duodenum Proximal Lesion & Exam. U.G.I. Tract Endoscopic Fibreoptic
G43.-	Extirpation Duodenum Proximal Lesion & Exam. U.G.I. Tract Endoscopic NEC
D02.-	Extirpation Ear External Lesion
D02.-	Extirpation Ear External Skin Lesion
D19.-	Extirpation Ear Middle Lesion
Q17.-	Extirpation Endometrium Endoscopic
C12.-	Extirpation Eyelid Lesion
C12.-	Extirpation Eyelid Skin Lesion
A38.5	Extirpation Falx Cerebri Lesion
T53.-	Extirpation Fascia Lesion
G43.-	Extirpation Gastrointestinal Tract Upper Lesion Endoscopic Fibreoptic
G42.-	Extirpation Gastrointestinal Tract Upper Lesion Endoscopic Fibreoptic Other
G43.-	Extirpation Gastrointestinal Tract Upper Lesion Endoscopic NEC
G42.-	Extirpation Gastrointestinal Tract Upper Lesion Endoscopic Other NEC
G79.1	Extirpation Ileum Lesion Endoscopic
G70.-	Extirpation Ileum Lesion Open
G79.1	Extirpation Intestine Small Lesion Endoscopic NEC
G70.-	Extirpation Intestine Small Lesion Open NEC
G64.1	Extirpation Jejunum Lesion Endoscopic
G59.-	Extirpation Jejunum Lesion Open
M10.1	Extirpation Kidney Lesion Endoscopic
M04.-	Extirpation Kidney Lesion Open
E30.-	Extirpation Larynx Lesion Open
	Extirpation Lesion – see Extirpation site Lesion
F02.-	Extirpation Lip Lesion
F02.-	Extirpation Lip Mucosa Lesion
F02.-	Extirpation Lip Skin Lesion
J03.-	Extirpation Liver Lesion
E55.-	Extirpation Lung Lesion Open
E62.1	Extirpation Mediastinum Lesion Endoscopic
A43.1	Extirpation Meninges Skull Base Lesion
A43.2	Extirpation Meninges Skull Clivus Lesion
F38.-	Extirpation Mouth Lesion NEC

S64.-	Extirpation Nail Bed
E64.1	Extirpation Nasal Cavity Lesion Endoscopic
E24.1	Extirpation Nasopharynx Lesion Endoscopic
	Extirpation Nerve – see also Destruction Nerve
	Extirpation Nerve – see also Transection Nerve
A28.-	Extirpation Nerve Cranial Extracranial NEC
A61.-	Extirpation Nerve Peripheral Lesion
A57.1	Extirpation Nerve Root Spinal Lesion
A27.-	Extirpation Nerve Vagus (x)
B35.3	Extirpation Nipple Lesion
B35.3	Extirpation Nipple Skin Lesion
E08.2	Extirpation Nose Internal Lesion NEC
G43.-	Extirpation Oesophagus Lesion & Exam. U.G.I. Tract Endoscopic Fibreoptic
G43.-	Extirpation Oesophagus Lesion & Exam. U.G.I. Tract Endoscopic NEC
G14.-	Extirpation Oesophagus Lesion Endoscopic Fibreoptic
G14.-	Extirpation Oesophagus Lesion Endoscopic NEC
G17.-	Extirpation Oesophagus Lesion Endoscopic Rigid
G04.-	Extirpation Oesophagus Lesion Open
C02.-	Extirpation Orbit Lesion
X53.-	Extirpation Organ Unspecified
Q49.1	Extirpation Ovary Lesion Access Minimal
Q49.1	Extirpation Ovary Lesion Endoscopic
F28.-	Extirpation Palate Lesion
J58.-	Extirpation Pancreas Lesion
N27.-	Extirpation Penis Lesion
N27.-	Extirpation Penis Skin Lesion
P11.-	Extirpation Perineum Female Lesion
P11.-	Extirpation Perineum Skin Female Lesion
T33.-	Extirpation Peritoneum Lesion Open
E24.2	Extirpation Pharynx Lesion Endoscopic
T10.1	Extirpation Pleura Lesion Access Minimal
T10.1	Extirpation Pleura Lesion Endoscopic
M62.1	Extirpation Prostate Lesion Open
G43.-	Extirpation Pylorus Lesion Endoscopic Fibreoptic
G43.-	Extirpation Pylorus Lesion Endoscopic NEC
H23.-	Extirpation Rectum Lesion Endoscopic NEC
H34.-	Extirpation Rectum Lesion Open
H23.-	Extirpation Rectum Lesion Sigmoidoscope Fibreoptic
H26.-	Extirpation Rectum Lesion Sigmoidoscope Rigid
F45.-	Extirpation Salivary Gland Lesion
C53.-	Extirpation Sclera Lesion
N01.-	Extirpation Scrotum
N01.-	Extirpation Scrotum Skin
A44.2	Extirpation Spinal Cord Lesion NEC
A51.1	Extirpation Spinal Cord Meninges Lesion
A44.-	Extirpation Spinal Cord Partial
V43.-	Extirpation Spine Lesion
G43.-	Extirpation Stomach Lesion Endoscopic Fibreoptic
G43.-	Extirpation Stomach Lesion Endoscopic NEC
G17.-	Extirpation Stomach Lesion Gastroscope Rigid

G29.-	Extirpation Stomach Lesion Open
A38.6	Extirpation Tentorium Cerebelli Lesion
N07.-	Extirpation Testis Lesion
F23.-	Extirpation Tongue Lesion
T29.3	Extirpation Umbilicus Lesion
M29.1	Extirpation Ureter Lesion Endoscopic
M32.1	Extirpation Ureteric Orifice Lesion Endoscopic
M76.1	Extirpation Urethra Lesion Endoscopic
M81.1	Extirpation Urethra Meatus Lesion
P20.-	Extirpation Vagina Lesion
P06.-	Extirpation Vulva Lesion
P06.-	Extirpation Vulva Skin Lesion
X58.1	Extracorporeal Membrane Oxygenation
	Extraction – see also Delivery
	Extraction – see also Removal from site
W36.5	Extraction Bone Marrow Diagnostic NEC
B37.3	Extraction Breast Milk
C71.-	Extraction Cataract Extracapsular
C72.-	Extraction Cataract Intracapsular
C74.-	Extraction Cataract NEC
C71.-	Extraction Lens Extracapsular
C72.1	Extraction Lens Forceps
C72.-	Extraction Lens Intracapsular
C71.1	Extraction Lens Linear Simple
C74.-	Extraction Lens NEC
C72.2	Extraction Lens Suction
Q11.4	Extraction Menses
N34.6	Extraction Sperm Testicular
F51.2	Extraction Submandibular Duct Calculus Open
F10.-	Extraction Tooth Multiple
F10.-	Extraction Tooth Simple
F10.-	Extraction Tooth Single
F09.-	Extraction Tooth Wisdom
M75.4	Extraction Urethral Calculus Open
C69.-	Eye Anterior Chamber Operations NEC
Z18.-	Eye Anterior Chamber site
Z16.-	Eye External Structure site
C31.-	Eye Muscle Operations Combined
C37.-	Eye Muscle Operations NEC
Z17.-	Eye Muscle site NEC
C86.-	Eye Operations NEC
Z19.-	Eye site NEC
Z17.-	Eye Tendon site NEC
C61.-	Eye Trabecular Meshwork Operations NEC
C10.-	Eyebrow Operations
Z16.2	Eyebrow site
C10.-	Eyebrow Skin Operations
Z16.2	Eyebrow Skin site
C23.-	Eyelid Operations
C22.-	Eyelid Operations Other NEC

Z16.4	Eyelid site
C23.-	Eyelid Skin Operations
C22.-	Eyelid Skin Operations Other NEC
Z16.4	Eyelid Skin site

F

S01.-	Facelift
V67.1	Facetectomy Spine Lumbar Medial Posterior
V68.1	Facetectomy Spine Lumbar Medial Posterior Revisional
Y73.-	Facilitating Operations NOC
Y71.4	Failed Minimal Access Approach Converted to Open
	Failed Operations – refer to Tabular List Introduction
Y71.5	Failed Percutaneous Approach Converted to Open
Q38.-	Fallopian Tube Operations Endoscopic Therapeutic NEC
Q41.-	Fallopian Tube Operations NEC
Q34.-	Fallopian Tube Operations Open NEC
Q41.5	Fallopian Tube Operations Patency NEC
Z46.2	Fallopian Tube site
Q39.9	Falloposcopy NEC
T57.-	Fascia Operations NEC
Z62.1	Fascia site
T52.-	Fasciectomy
T54.-	Fasciotomy
T55.-	Fasciotomy Release
Z76.-	Femur site
W18.1	Fenestration Bone Cortex
	Fenestration Disc Intervertebral – see Excision Disc Intervertebral
E13.8	Fenestration Maxillary
X55.3	Fenestration Organ Unspecified
K69.2	Fenestration Pericardium
T08.-	Fenestration Pleura
K14.2	Fenestration Septum Atrial
K16.-	Fenestration Septum Atrial Transluminal Percutaneous
Y96.-	Fertilisation In Vitro
Q56.1	Fertility Investigation Female NEC
Q41.-	Fertility Investigation Female Tubal Patency
N34.1	Fertility Investigation Male NEC
Q56.2	Fertiloscopy
R06.2	Feticide NEC
R06.1	Feticide Selective
R02.-	Fetoscopy
R01.-	Fetus Operations Therapeutic Endoscopic
R04.-	Fetus Operations Therapeutic Percutaneous
Z45.3	Fetus site
H25.-	Fibrosigmoidoscopy
Z78.1	Fibula & Tibia Shaft Combination site

Z78.-	Fibula site NEC
L79.1	Filter Vena Cava Insertion
C60.-	Filtering Iris
Q32.-	Fimbria Operations
Z46.1	Fimbria site
H55.-	Fistula Anal Operations NEC
O05.-	Fistula Arteriovenous Dural Operations (L)
M37.5	Fistula Bladder Repair NEC
M62.4	Fistula Rectoprostatic Repair
L74.2	Fistulisation Arteriovenous Dialysis
L74.2	Fistulisation Arteriovenous NEC
L74.6	Fistulisation Graft Dialysis
G08.2	Fistulisation Oesophagus External NEC
M54.1	Fistulisation Urethrovaginal
M41.2	Fistulisation Vesicovaginal
Y39.1	Fistulogram NOC
H55.5	Fistulography Anal Fistula
L74.-	Fistulography Arteriovenous Fistula
F15.2	Fitting Bracket Orthodontic
V04.1	Fitting Cranioplasty Bands Dynamic
F63.2	Fitting Denture or Obturator
F15.3	Fitting Headgear Orthodontic
D13.6	Fitting Hearing Prosthesis External to Bone Anchored Fixtures
F15.4	Fitting Separators Orthodontic
F17.7	Fitting Teeth Bridge
F17.3	Fitting Tooth Crown Dental
W20.-	Fixation Bone & Reduction Fracture Open NEC
W19.-	Fixation Bone & Reduction Fragment Open
W30.-	Fixation Bone External
W25.-	Fixation Bone External & Reduction Fracture Closed
W25.3	Fixation Bone External & Remanipulation Fracture
W25.-	Fixation Bone Fracture External NEC
W24.-	Fixation Bone Fracture Internal NEC
W21.-	Fixation Bone Fracture Intra-articular Primary
W24.6	Fixation Bone Fracture Nail or Screw & Reduction Fracture Closed
W28.-	Fixation Bone Internal
W24.-	Fixation Bone Internal & Reduction Fracture Closed
W19.-	Fixation Bone Intramedullary & Reduction Fracture Open
W30.-	Fixation Bone NEC
C08.3	Fixation Bone Orbit Fracture Removal
W24.5	Fixation Bone Screw & Reduction Fragment Closed
H19.2	Fixation Caecum
W83.2	Fixation Cartilage Articular Lesion Endoscopic
H19.2	Fixation Colon
W27.-	Fixation Epiphysis
W27.5	Fixation Epiphysis Temporary
V11.-	Fixation Face
C60.3	Fixation Iris
V17.-	Fixation Jaw NEC
V17.-	Fixation Mandible

V11.-	Fixation Maxilla
C08.5	Fixation Orbit Fracture
C08.3	Fixation Orbit Removal
Q45.2	Fixation Ovary NEC
H35.-	Fixation Rectum Prolapse NEC
C85.-	Fixation Retina
V46.-	Fixation Spine Fracture
N13.2	Fixation Testis
P24.7	Fixation Vagina Sacrospinous
	Fixator – see Fixation
E11.-	Fixture Nose Prosthesis Operations
	Flap Bone – see also Flap site
E14.5	Flap Bone Ethmoid Sinus
E14.5	Flap Bone Frontal Sinus
E14.5	Flap Ethmoid Sinus Bone
C10.2	Flap Eyebrow Hair Bearing
C14.1	Flap Eyelid Skin
S18.-	Flap Fasciocutaneous Distant
S25.-	Flap Fasciocutaneous Local
E14.5	Flap Frontal Sinus Bone
S28.-	Flap Mucosa
T76.1	Flap Muscle Transfer Free Tissue Microvascular
S17.-	Flap Myocutaneous Distant
S24.-	Flap Myocutaneous Local
T36.5	Flap Omental Creation
	Flap Skin – see also Flap site
S18.-	Flap Skin & Fascia Distant
S25.-	Flap Skin & Fascia Local
S17.-	Flap Skin & Muscle Distant
S24.-	Flap Skin & Muscle Local
S20.-	Flap Skin Distant NEC
S19.-	Flap Skin Distant Pedicle
S21.-	Flap Skin Hair Bearing
S30.-	Flap Skin Head Operations NEC
S27.-	Flap Skin Local NEC
S26.-	Flap Skin Local Subcutaneous Pedicle
S27.-	Flap Skin NEC
S30.-	Flap Skin Neck Operations NEC
S31.-	Flap Skin Operations NEC
S23.-	Flap Skin Operations Relax Contracture
S22.-	Flap Skin Sensory
S28.1	Flap Tongue
Y53.4	Fluoroscopic Control Approach
Y03.1	Flushing Catheter NOC
W71.3	Forage Joint
V56.-	Foraminoplasty Spine NEC
V56.-	Foraminoplasty Spine Primary
V57.-	Foraminoplasty Spine Revisional
V22.3	Foraminotomy Spine Cervical NEC
V23.3	Foraminotomy Spine Cervical Revisional

V25.6	Foraminotomy Spine Lumbar Lateral NEC
V26.6	Foraminotomy Spine Lumbar Lateral Revisional
W11.-	Fracture Bone Surgical NEC
W10.-	Fracture Bone Surgical Open
N28.6	Fracture Penis Repair
	Fragmentation – see also Dissolution
	Fragmentation – see also Lithotripsy
J41.3	Fragmentation Bile Duct Calculus Endoscopic Retrograde
J52.1	Fragmentation Bile Duct Calculus Extracorporeal
J26.1	Fragmentation Gall Bladder Calculus Extracorporeal
J24.2	Fragmentation Gall Bladder Calculus Percutaneous
M09.-	Fragmentation Kidney Calculus Endoscopic NEC
M14.-	Fragmentation Kidney Calculus Extracorporeal
M09.-	Fragmentation Kidney Calculus Percutaneous NEC
M09.-	Fragmentation Kidney Calculus Percutaneous Nephroscopic
J68.1	Fragmentation Pancreas Calculus Extracorporeal
M28.-	Fragmentation Ureter Calculus Endoscopic NEC
M31.-	Fragmentation Ureter Calculus Extracorporeal
M26.-	Fragmentation Ureter Calculus Nephroscopic
M27.-	Fragmentation Ureter Calculus Ureteroscopic
Y18.1	Freeing Adhesions NOC
T42.3	Freeing Bowel Adhesions Endoscopic
T41.5	Freeing Bowel Adhesions Extensive
T41.3	Freeing Bowel Adhesions Limited
C43.1	Freeing Conjunctiva Adhesions
D17.3	Freeing Ear Ossicle Adhesions
C37.2	Freeing Eye Muscle Adhesions
Q38.1	Freeing Fallopian Tube Adhesions Access Minimal
Q38.1	Freeing Fallopian Tube Adhesions Endoscopic
Q34.1	Freeing Fallopian Tube Adhesions Open
T57.1	Freeing Fascia Adhesions
M08.8	Freeing Kidney Adhesions
F06.1	Freeing Lip Adhesions
T42.3	Freeing Mesentery Adhesions Endoscopic
T41.3	Freeing Mesentery Adhesions NEC
C37.2	Freeing Muscle Eye Adhesions
A73.2	Freeing Nerve Peripheral Adhesions NEC
E08.4	Freeing Nose Internal Adhesions
E04.4	Freeing Nose Turbinate Adhesions
Q49.2	Freeing Ovary Adhesions Access Minimal
Q49.2	Freeing Ovary Adhesions Endoscopic
Q47.2	Freeing Ovary Adhesions Open
K69.1	Freeing Pericardium Adhesions
T42.3	Freeing Peritoneum Adhesions Access Minimal
T42.3	Freeing Peritoneum Adhesions Endoscopic
T41.3	Freeing Peritoneum Adhesions NEC
N30.2	Freeing Prepuce Adhesions
A51.2	Freeing Spinal Cord Meninges Adhesions
A49.4	Freeing Spinal Tether Complex
A49.1	Freeing Spinal Tether NEC

T69.-	Freeing Tendon
F26.4	Freeing Tongue Adhesions
Q20.1	Freeing Uterus Adhesions
P29.1	Freeing Vagina Adhesions
F05.1	Frenectomy Lip
F42.3	Frenectomy NEC
F26.2	Frenectomy Tongue
F26.3	Frenotomy Tongue
N28.4	Frenuloplasty Penis
E14.-	Frontal Sinus Operations Endoscopic Diagnostic
E14.-	Frontal Sinus Operations NEC
Z23.2	Frontal Sinus site
E14.1	Frontoethmoidectomy External
X61.1	Functional Therapy Session
G24.-	Fundoplication Antireflux NEC
G25.1	Fundoplication Stomach Revision
W61.-	Fusion Joint & Graft Bone Articular NEC
W60.-	Fusion Joint & Graft Bone NEC
V37.4	Fusion Joint Atlanto-occipital
V66.1	Fusion Joint Atlanto-occipital Revisional
V37.-	Fusion Joint Atlantoaxial NEC
V37.6	Fusion Joint Atlantoaxial Posterior Pedicle Screw
V66.3	Fusion Joint Atlantoaxial Posterior Pedicle Screw Revisional
V66.4	Fusion Joint Atlantoaxial Posterior Revisional NEC
V37.5	Fusion Joint Atlantoaxial Posterior Transarticular Screw
V66.2	Fusion Joint Atlantoaxial Posterior Transarticular Screw Revisional
W64.-	Fusion Joint Conversion NEC
W04.-	Fusion Joint Hindfoot
W03.-	Fusion Joint Interphalangeal
W59.-	Fusion Joint Interphalangeal Toe
W59.-	Fusion Joint Metatarsophalangeal First
W03.5	Fusion Joint Midfoot Forefoot Localised
W62.-	Fusion Joint NEC
W63.-	Fusion Joint Revisional NEC
V37.-	Fusion Joint Spine Cervical NEC
V39.1	Fusion Joint Spine Cervical Revisional
V38.-	Fusion Joint Spine Lumbar NEC
V39.-	Fusion Joint Spine Lumbar Revisional
V38.-	Fusion Joint Spine NEC
V39.-	Fusion Joint Spine Revisional
V38.1	Fusion Joint Spine Thoracic NEC
V39.2	Fusion Joint Spine Thoracic Revisional
W59.-	Fusion Joint Toe
V37.7	Fusion Junction Occipitocervical NEC
V66.1	Fusion Junction Occipitocervical Revisional
V40.2	Fusion Spine Cervical Instrumented Posterior NEC
V40.4	Fusion Spine Lumbar Instrumented Posterior NEC
V40.3	Fusion Spine Thoracic Instrumented Posterior NEC

G

J08.-	Gall Bladder Operations Endoscopic Therapeutic
J08.-	Gall Bladder Operations Laparoscopic
J26.-	Gall Bladder Operations NEC
J23.-	Gall Bladder Operations Open NEC
J25.-	Gall Bladder Operations Percutaneous Diagnostic
J24.-	Gall Bladder Operations Percutaneous Therapeutic
J08.-	Gall Bladder Operations Peritoneoscope
Z30.2	Gall Bladder site
Q38.3	Gametes Intrafallopian Transfer Endoscopic
Q13.-	Gametes Uterine Cavity Introduction
T61.-	Ganglion Operations
G28.-	Gastrectomy NEC
G28.-	Gastrectomy Partial
G28.5	Gastrectomy Sleeve
G27.-	Gastrectomy Total
G48.-	Gastric Bubble
O11.1	Gastro-oesophageal Junction site (Z)
G49.1	Gastroduodenectomy
G31.-	Gastroduodenostomy
G33.-	Gastroenterostomy
Y51.-	Gastrointestinal Tract Approach Opening Artificial
G46.-	Gastrointestinal Tract Upper Operations Endoscopic Therapeutic NEC
G44.-	Gastrointestinal Tract Upper Operations Endoscopic Therapeutic Other NEC
G46.-	Gastrointestinal Tract Upper Operations Therapeutic Fibreoptic NEC
G44.-	Gastrointestinal Tract Upper Operations Therapeutic Fibreoptic Other NEC
G33.1	Gastrojejunostomy NEC
G24.4	Gastropexy Antireflux
G36.1	Gastropexy NEC
G24.5	Gastroplasty & Antireflux Operations HFQ
G30.1	Gastroplasty NEC
G45.-	Gastroscopy Fibreoptic
G45.-	Gastroscopy NEC
G19.-	Gastroscopy Rigid
Y51.2	Gastrostomy Approach
G44.-	Gastrostomy Endoscopic Fibreoptic Percutaneous
G34.-	Gastrostomy NEC
G38.5	Gastrotomy NEC
V19.2	Genioplasty Jaw NEC
V19.2	Genioplasty Mandible
Z43.-	Genital Organ Male site

Q56.-	Genital Tract Female Operations NEC
Z46.-	Genital Tract Female site NEC
N34.-	Genital Tract Male Operations NEC
N35.-	Genitalia Male Non-operative Interventions
Y95.-	Gestational Age
F20.-	Gingiva Operations
Z25.4	Gingiva site
F20.-	Gingivectomy
F20.4	Gingivoplasty
C65.-	Glaucoma Operations Following Surgery
U26.1	Glomerular Filtration Rate Testing
F22.-	Glossectomy
F24.3	Glossotomy
C47.4	Gluing Cornea
C61.4	Goniopuncture
C61.3	Goniotomy
H57.-	Graciloplasty Dynamic Sphincter
H57.4	Graciloplasty Sphincter
E02.7	Graft Alar Reconstruction Cartilage
	Graft Artery – see Anastomosis Artery
	Graft Artery – see Bypass Artery
	Graft Artery – see Reconstruction Artery
	Graft Artery – see Repair Artery
	Graft Artery – see Replacement Artery
	Graft Bone – see also Autograft Bone
W60.-	Graft Bone & Fusion Joint NEC
W61.-	Graft Bone Articular & Fusion Joint NEC
V05.5	Graft Bone Cranium
W34.-	Graft Bone Marrow
W32.-	Graft Bone NEC
V54.2	Graft Bone Spine NEC
W32.4	Graft Bone Synthetic
C11.5	Graft Canthus Skin
C40.-	Graft Conjunctiva
C46.-	Graft Cornea
C46.6	Graft Cornea Amniotic Membrane
C44.3	Graft Cornea Endothelial
C46.5	Graft Cornea Lamellar Deep
C46.2	Graft Cornea Lamellar NEC
C46.3	Graft Cornea Penetrating
C46.8	Graft Cornea Revision
D22.1	Graft Eustachian Canal
C10.3	Graft Eyebrow Hair Bearing
C14.3	Graft Eyelid Cartilage
C14.5	Graft Eyelid Fascia
C14.2	Graft Eyelid Skin
C14.4	Graft Eyelid Skin & Fat
V19.3	Graft Jaw Alveolar NEC
V19.3	Graft Mandible Alveolar
V13.2	Graft Maxilla Alveolar

F40.-	Graft Mouth NEC
S38.-	Graft Mucosa
A24.-	Graft Nerve Cranial Microsurgical
A24.-	Graft Nerve Cranial NEC
A62.-	Graft Nerve Peripheral Microsurgical
A62.6	Graft Nerve Peripheral Multiple Microsurgical NEC
A63.-	Graft Nerve Peripheral NEC
Y27.-	Graft NOC
D16.2	Graft Ossicular Chain
N28.7	Graft Penis
Y27.6	Graft Prosthetic NOC
C57.3	Graft Sclera
E03.7	Graft Septal Reconstruction
S34.-	Graft Skin Hair Bearing NEC
S33.-	Graft Skin Hair Bearing Scalp
S37.-	Graft Skin NEC
S36.-	Graft Skin Pinch
S35.-	Graft Skin Split
S39.-	Graft Skin Tissue NEC
V42.3	Graft Spine & Release Anterolateral
W99.-	Graft Stem Cells Cord Blood to Bone Marrow
S39.-	Graft Subcutaneous Tissue NEC
L93.5	Graft Vein
L83.1	Graft Vein Saphenous Crossover
D20.-	Grommet Tympanic Membrane Attention
D15.1	Grommet Tympanic Membrane Insertion
	Guidance – see Education
Z01.7	Gyrus Cingulate site

H

X43.1	Haemodialysis Albumin Extracorporeal
X40.3	Haemodialysis NEC
X40.4	Haemofiltration
X40.7	Haemoperfusion
H53.-	Haemorrhoid Operations NEC
H51.-	Haemorrhoidectomy
H51.3	Haemorrhoidectomy Stapled
	Haemostasis – see also Arrest Bleeding site Postoperative Surgical
	Haemostasis – see also Packing site
H21.-	Haemostasis Caecum Endoscopic Fibreoptic
H21.-	Haemostasis Caecum Endoscopic NEC
H21.-	Haemostasis Colon Endoscopic Fibreoptic NEC
H21.-	Haemostasis Colon Endoscopic NEC
H24.2	Haemostasis Lower Bowel Sigmoidoscope Fibreoptic
E05.-	Haemostasis Nose Internal
Y66.-	Harvest Bone
Y66.7	Harvest Bone Marrow
Y69.-	Harvest Cartilage
Y67.1	Harvest Cartilage & Skin Composite Ear
W89.2	Harvest Chondrocytes Autologous Endoscopic
Y67.2	Harvest Dermis Fat
Y59.-	Harvest Fascia & Skin Flap
Y60.-	Harvest Fascia Lata
Y60.-	Harvest Fascia NEC
Y60.-	Harvest Fascia Sheet
Y62.-	Harvest Muscle & Skin Flap NEC
Y61.-	Harvest Muscle & Skin Flap Trunk
Y64.-	Harvest Muscle Flap NEC
Y63.-	Harvest Muscle Flap Trunk
Y54.-	Harvest Nerve
Y69.1	Harvest Omentum
Y67.1	Harvest Skin & Cartilage Composite Ear
Y59.-	Harvest Skin & Fascia Flap
Y67.2	Harvest Skin & Fat Composite
Y62.-	Harvest Skin & Muscle Flap NEC
Y61.-	Harvest Skin & Muscle Flap Trunk
Y55.-	Harvest Skin Flap Limb Pattern Random
Y57.-	Harvest Skin Flap Pattern Axial
Y56.-	Harvest Skin Flap Pattern Random NEC
Y58.1	Harvest Skin Flap Post Auricular

Y58.-	Harvest Skin Graft NEC
Y65.-	Harvest Tendon
Y67.-	Harvest Tissue Multiple NEC
Y69.-	Harvest Tissue NEC
Y69.3	Harvest Vein
K54.-	Heart Assist Operations Open
K56.-	Heart Assist Operations Transluminal
K56.-	Heart Assist System Transluminal
K52.-	Heart Conducting System Operations Open
K58.-	Heart Conducting System Study
K66.-	Heart Operations NEC
K55.-	Heart Operations Open NEC
K58.-	Heart Operations Transluminal Diagnostic
K62.-	Heart Operations Transluminal Therapeutic NEC
K57.-	Heart Operations Transluminal Therapeutic Other NEC
K15.-	Heart Septum Operations Closed
K14.-	Heart Septum Operations Open NEC
K16.-	Heart Septum Operations Transluminal Therapeutic
Z33.-	Heart site NEC
K34.-	Heart Valve Operations Open NEC
K35.-	Heart Valve Operations Transluminal Therapeutic
Z32.-	Heart Valve site
K38.-	Heart Valve Structure Adjacent Operations NEC
Z33.2	Heart Ventricle Septum site
K23.-	Heart Wall Operations NEC
Z33.3	Heart Wall site
	Hemiarthroplasty – see also Arthroplasty
W52.-	Hemiarthroplasty Bone Articulation Prosthetic Cemented NEC
W54.-	Hemiarthroplasty Bone Articulation Prosthetic NEC
W53.-	Hemiarthroplasty Bone Articulation Prosthetic Uncemented NEC
W46.-	Hemiarthroplasty Femur Head Prosthetic Cemented
W48.-	Hemiarthroplasty Femur Head Prosthetic NEC
W47.-	Hemiarthroplasty Femur Head Prosthetic Uncemented
W49.-	Hemiarthroplasty Humerus Head Prosthetic Cemented
W51.-	Hemiarthroplasty Humerus Head Prosthetic NEC
W50.-	Hemiarthroplasty Humerus Head Prosthetic Uncemented
O24.-	Hemiarthroplasty Radius Head Prosthetic Cemented (W)
O26.-	Hemiarthroplasty Radius Head Prosthetic NEC (W)
O25.-	Hemiarthroplasty Radius Head Prosthetic Uncemented (W)
H09.-	Hemicolectomy Left
H11.-	Hemicolectomy NEC
H06.-	Hemicolectomy Right Extended
H07.-	Hemicolectomy Right NEC
V05.7	Hemicraniotomy
J02.-	Hemihepatectomy
	Hemilaminectomy – see also Laminectomy
V67.2	Hemilaminectomy Spine Lumbar
V68.2	Hemilaminectomy Spine Lumbar Revisional
V14.1	Hemimandibulectomy
M03.1	Heminephrectomy Kidney Duplex

A01.1	Hemispherectomy
B08.3	Hemithyroidectomy
Z30.4	Hepatic Duct site
O30.1	Hepatic Flexure site (Z)
	Herniorrhaphy – see also Repair Hernia
T27.-	Herniorrhaphy Abdominal Wall NEC
T22.-	Herniorrhaphy Femoral NEC
T25.-	Herniorrhaphy Incisional NEC
T20.-	Herniorrhaphy Inguinal NEC
T25.-	Herniorrhaphy Parastomal NEC
T24.-	Herniorrhaphy Umbilical
T27.-	Herniorrhaphy Ventral
T19.-	Herniotomy
X97.-	High Cost Anaesthesia Drugs
X86.-	High Cost Anti-infective Drugs
X83.-	High Cost Cardiovascular Drugs
X95.-	High Cost Dermatology Drugs
X98.-	High Cost Drugs Other
X94.-	High Cost Ear Nose & Throat Drugs
X87.-	High Cost Endocrinology Drugs
X81.-	High Cost Gastrointestinal Drugs
X90.-	High Cost Haematology & Nutrition Drugs
X82.-	High Cost Hypertensive Drugs
X96.-	High Cost Immunology Drugs
X89.-	High Cost Immunosuppressant Drugs
X91.-	High Cost Metabolic Drugs
X92.-	High Cost Musculoskeletal Drugs
X85.-	High Cost Neurology Drugs
X93.-	High Cost Ophthalmology Drugs
X88.-	High Cost Reproductive & Urinary Tract Drugs
X84.-	High Cost Respiratory Drugs
Z69.-	Humerus site
N11.-	Hydrocele Sac Operations
Q41.2	Hydrotubation Fallopian Tube
P15.1	Hymenectomy
P15.4	Hymenotomy
X52.1	Hyperbaric Therapy
B01.-	Hypophysectomy
X51.1	Hypothermia Therapy
Q07.-	Hysterectomy Abdominal
R25.1	Hysterectomy Caesarean
Q07.-	Hysterectomy NEC
Q08.-	Hysterectomy Vaginal
Q07.-	Hysterocolpectomy Abdominal
Q08.-	Hysterocolpectomy Vaginal
Q54.6	Hysteropexy Infracoccygeal
Q41.1	Hysterosalpingography
Q18.-	Hysteroscopy
U09.2	Hysterosonography
Q09.-	Hysterotomy
Q09.6	Hysterotomy NEC

I

G69.-	Ileectomy
H68.-	Ileoanal Pouch Operations Diagnostic
H66.-	Ileoanal Pouch Operations Therapeutic
M36.2	Ileocystoplasty
G80.-	Ileoscopy
H09.4	Ileostomy & Excision Colon Left
H11.4	Ileostomy & Excision Colon NEC
H07.4	Ileostomy & Excision Colon Right
H06.4	Ileostomy & Excision Colon Right Extended
H10.4	Ileostomy & Excision Colon Sigmoid
H05.-	Ileostomy & Excision Colon Total
H08.4	Ileostomy & Excision Colon Transverse
H04.1	Ileostomy & Panproctocolectomy
Y51.3	Ileostomy Approach
G75.3	Ileostomy Closure
G74.-	Ileostomy Creation
G75.5	Ileostomy Prolapse Reduction
G75.2	Ileostomy Prolapse Repair
G75.1	Ileostomy Refashioning
G75.6	Ileostomy Resiting
G79.-	Ileum Operations Endoscopic Therapeutic
G82.-	Ileum Operations NEC
G78.-	Ileum Operations Open NEC
Z27.6	Ileum site
Z75.3	Ilium Wing site
Y53.-	Image Control Approach
Y53.5	Image Intensifier Control Approach NEC
	Imaging – see also Scan
U08.-	Imaging Abdomen Diagnostic
U08.5	Imaging Abdomen Magnetic Resonance
U11.7	Imaging Angiography Magnetic Resonance
U01.2	Imaging Body Whole Magnetic Resonance
U01.-	Imaging Body Whole NEC
U13.3	Imaging Bone Magnetic Resonance
U05.2	Imaging Brain Magnetic Resonance
U05.3	Imaging Brain Magnetic Resonance Functional
U18.-	Imaging Breast Diagnostic
U10.3	Imaging Cardiac Magnetic Resonance
U05.-	Imaging Central Nervous Diagnostic
U07.-	Imaging Chest Diagnostic

U07.2	Imaging Chest Magnetic Resonance
U04.-	Imaging Dental
U21.-	Imaging Diagnostic NEC
U36.-	Imaging Diagnostic Other NEC
Y94.4	Imaging Diethylenetriamine Pentacetic Acid
U17.-	Imaging Digestive Tract
Y94.1	Imaging Dopamine Transporter Scan
U06.-	Imaging Face Neck Diagnostic
Y93.-	Imaging Gallium-67
U08.4	Imaging Gastrointestinal Upper Series
U12.-	Imaging Genitourinary System Diagnostic
U37.-	Imaging Genitourinary System Diagnostic Other
U05.2	Imaging Head Magnetic Resonance
U05.3	Imaging Head Magnetic Resonance Functional
U10.-	Imaging Heart Diagnostic
U16.-	Imaging Hepatobiliary System
U13.3	Imaging Joint Magnetic Resonance
U37.1	Imaging Kidney Magnetic Resonance
Y94.3	Imaging Metaiodobenzylguanidine
U13.-	Imaging Musculoskeletal System Diagnostic
Y94.2	Imaging Octreotide
U09.-	Imaging Pelvis Diagnostic
U09.3	Imaging Pelvis Magnetic Resonance
Y94.-	Imaging Radiopharmaceutical
U15.-	Imaging Respiratory System
C87.1	Imaging Retina Digital
U05.5	Imaging Spinal Cord Magnetic Resonance
U05.5	Imaging Spine Magnetic Resonance
U11.-	Imaging Vascular System Diagnostic
U35.-	Imaging Vascular System Diagnostic Other
U11.7	Imaging Venography Magnetic Resonance
C54.2	Imbrication Sclera
Y70.2	Immediate Operations NOC
	Immobilisation – see also Support
X48.-	Immobilisation Plaster Cast
X37.3	Immunotherapy Intramuscular
X35.3	Immunotherapy Intravenous
X38.4	Immunotherapy Subcutaneous
	Implant – see also Implantation
C04.-	Implant Orbit Attention
C03.-	Implant Orbit Insertion
C54.6	Implant Sclera Removal
	Implantation – see also Transfer
L03.2	Implantation Arterial Duct Stent Transluminal Percutaneous
K46.-	Implantation Artery Mammary Heart
K46.-	Implantation Artery Thoracic Heart
W71.4	Implantation Articular Structure Chondrocyte Autologous Open
M55.2	Implantation Bladder Outlet Female Urinary Sphincter Artificial
M64.2	Implantation Bladder Outlet Male Urinary Sphincter Artificial
W05.3	Implantation Bone Endoprosthesis

W05.2	Implantation Bone Endoprosthesis Massive
A09.1	Implantation Brainstem Auditory Implant
K59.-	Implantation Cardioverter Defibrillator
K72.1	Implantation Cardioverter Defibrillator Subcutaneous
K59.6	Implantation Cardioverter Defibrillator Three Electrode Leads
U19.1	Implantation Electrocardiography Loop Recorder
A54.3	Implantation Intrathecal Drug Delivery Device Adjacent Spinal Cord
F11.-	Implantation Jaw
W85.3	Implantation Joint Knee Chondrocyte Autologous
	Implantation Neurostimulator – see Neurostimulator site
K61.7	Implantation Pacemaker Cardiac Biventricular
K61.6	Implantation Pacemaker Cardiac Dual Chamber
K60.6	Implantation Pacemaker Cardiac Dual Chamber Intravenous
K60.1	Implantation Pacemaker Cardiac Intravenous NEC
K61.1	Implantation Pacemaker Cardiac NEC
K61.5	Implantation Pacemaker Cardiac Single Chamber
K60.5	Implantation Pacemaker Cardiac Single Chamber Intravenous
K61.1	Implantation Pacemaker Cardiac Sutureless Screw-in
T02.2	Implantation Pectus Excavatum Correction Silicone
B02.2	Implantation Pituitary Gland Substance Radioactive
M70.6	Implantation Prostate Seed Radioactive
M71.2	Implantation Prostate Substance Radioactive
	Implantation Prosthesis – see Prosthesis site
Y36.3	Implantation Seed Radioactive NOC
	Implantation Stent – see also Insertion site Stent
	Implantation Stimulator – see Stimulator site
	Implantation System – see System
F08.-	Implantation Tooth
Q13.1	Implantation Uterus Egg Fertilised
P20.5	Implantation Vagina Radioactive
K54.1	Implantation Ventricular Assist Device Open
P06.4	Implantation Vulva Radioactive
E85.3	Improvement Ventilation Efficiency
	Improving – see Improvement
Y96.-	In Vitro Fertilisation
U22.2	Inactivation Functional Brain Hemisphere Single Test
	Incision & Curettage – see Curettage
	Incision & Drainage – see Drainage
	Incision – see also Exploration
H56.3	Incision Anus Septum
K52.6	Incision Atria Tissue
D08.4	Incision Auditory Canal External
J33.-	Incision Bile Duct
M66.2	Incision Bladder Neck Male Endoscopic NEC
M56.2	Incision Bladder Outlet Female Endoscopic
M66.2	Incision Bladder Outlet Male Endoscopic
B33.-	Incision Breast
H16.-	Incision Caecum
H16.-	Incision Colon
C41.-	Incision Conjunctiva

C49.-	Incision Cornea
G53.5	Incision Duodenum NEC
D15.-	Incision Eardrum
C10.5	Incision Eyebrow Lesion
C10.5	Incision Eyebrow Skin Lesion
C19.-	Incision Eyelid
C19.-	Incision Eyelid Skin
Q31.-	Incision Fallopian Tube
J21.-	Incision Gall Bladder
K53.-	Incision Heart NEC
K32.-	Incision Heart Valve Closed
K31.-	Incision Heart Valve NEC
K31.-	Incision Heart Valve Open
P15.4	Incision Hymen
C62.-	Incision Iris
G63.2	Incision Jejunum
W81.4	Incision Joint NEC
M06.-	Incision Kidney
M06.-	Incision Kidney Pelvis
C24.5	Incision Lacrimal Gland
C26.4	Incision Lacrimal Sac
Y08.6	Incision Laser NOC
L87.6	Incision Leg Vein Varicose
C73.-	Incision Lens Capsule
Y30.1	Incision Lesion NOC
J05.-	Incision Liver
E57.4	Incision Lung NEC
F42.2	Incision Mouth NEC
S70.2	Incision Nail
S66.3	Incision Nail Bed
E27.3	Incision Nasopharynx NEC
Y30.-	Incision NOC
E03.5	Incision Nose Septum
G09.-	Incision Oesophagus
C06.-	Incision Orbit
X55.2	Incision Organ Unspecified
F32.3	Incision Palate
J62.-	Incision Pancreas
N32.3	Incision Penis NEC
K69.-	Incision Pericardium
N24.4	Incision Periurethral Tissue Male
E27.3	Incision Pharynx NEC
G40.-	Incision Pylorus
F46.-	Incision Salivary Gland
	Incision Scar – see Incision Skin Lesion
C55.-	Incision Sclera
N22.2	Incision Seminal Vesicle
S47.-	Incision Skin
J38.-	Incision Sphincter Oddi Endoscopic
J35.-	Incision Sphincter Oddi NEC

G38.5	Incision Stomach NEC
S47.-	Incision Subcutaneous Tissue
B10.4	Incision Thyroglossal Cyst
B12.3	Incision Thyroid Lesion
F24.-	Incision Tongue
F26.3	Incision Tongue Frenulum
M23.-	Incision Ureter
M32.5	Incision Ureterocele Endoscopic
Q09.6	Incision Uterus NEC
P14.-	Incision Vagina Introitus
L93.2	Incision Vein NEC
C60.2	Inclusion Iris
	Incomplete Operations – refer to Tabular List Introduction
G48.3	Induction Emesis
X35.1	Induction Labour Intravenous
R15.1	Induction Labour Medical
R15.1	Induction Labour Misoprostol
R15.-	Induction Labour NEC
R15.1	Induction Labour Oxytocin
R15.1	Induction Labour Prostaglandin
R14.-	Induction Labour Surgical
Q56.1	Infertility Investigation Female NEC
Q41.-	Infertility Investigation Female Tubal Patency
N34.1	Infertility Investigation Male NEC
S49.1	Inflation Expander Skin
S49.1	Inflation Expander Skin Breast
K37.-	Infundibulectomy Heart
X29.3	Infusion Fluids Subcutaneous
X29.1	Infusion Insulin Subcutaneous Pump
X29.-	Infusion Therapeutic Continuous
X28.-	Infusion Therapeutic Intermittent
X39.4	Inhalation Administration Therapeutic Substance
	Injection – see also Insertion
	Injection – see also Introduction
Q14.-	Injection Amniotic Cavity Prostaglandin
Y82.2	Injection Anaesthetic Local NEC
X30.6	Injection Anaesthetic NEC
X35.5	Injection Antimicrobial Therapy Intravenous
L74.7	Injection Arteriovenous Fistula Radiocontrast
K50.3	Injection Artery Coronary Transluminal Percutaneous NEC
M43.4	Injection Bladder Nerve Neurolytic Endoscopic
M56.3	Injection Bladder Outlet Female Inert Endoscopic
M66.3	Injection Bladder Outlet Male Inert Endoscopic
M49.5	Injection Bladder Wall Substance Therapeutic
C65.2	Injection Bleb Following Glaucoma Surgery
B37.2	Injection Breast
T62.5	Injection Bursa
A54.-	Injection Cerebrospinal Fluid
Y09.2	Injection Destructive NOC
D23.1	Injection Ear Inner Transtympanic

D20.7	Injection Ear Middle Transtympanic
Y81.-	Injection Epidural Anaesthetic
A52.-	Injection Epidural Therapeutic
C69.3	Injection Eye Anterior Chamber
C86.7	Injection Eye Around Therapeutic Substance
C89.3	Injection Eye Posterior Segment NEC
C89.2	Injection Eye Posterior Segment Steroid
C89.3	Injection Eye Posterior Segment Substance Therapeutic
C22.4	Injection Eyelid
Q38.2	Injection Fallopian Tube Access Minimal
Q38.2	Injection Fallopian Tube Endoscopic
Y39.1	Injection Fistula Radiocontrast NOC
G43.4	Injection G.I.Tract Upper Lesion Sclerosing Agent
G43.6	Injection G.I.Tract Upper Lesion Therapy Fibreoptic Endoscopic
T61.3	Injection Ganglion
F48.5	Injection Gland Salivary Therapeutic Substance
X30.-	Injection Globulin
H52.3	Injection Haemorrhoid NEC
H52.3	Injection Haemorrhoid Sclerosing
X38.3	Injection Hormone NEC
Y39.3	Injection Inert NOC
	Injection Intra-amniotic – see Injection Uterine Cavity
S53.-	Injection Intradermal NEC
X37.-	Injection Intramuscular NEC
A54.-	Injection Intrathecal
	Injection Intrauterine – see Injection Uterine Cavity
X35.-	Injection Intravenous NEC
W90.-	Injection Joint
M13.-	Injection Kidney Pelvis Percutaneous
M13.-	Injection Kidney Percutaneous
E38.1	Injection Larynx
L86.-	Injection Leg Vein Varicose
Y12.2	Injection Lesion Destructive NOC
Y12.1	Injection Lesion Sclerosing NOC
J10.3	Injection Liver Transluminal Percutaneous
M43.4	Injection Nerve Bladder Neurolytic Endoscopic
A60.5	Injection Nerve Peripheral Destructive
A73.5	Injection Nerve Peripheral Therapeutic
A57.4	Injection Nerve Root Spinal Destructive
A57.7	Injection Nerve Root Spinal Therapeutic
A81.2	Injection Nerve Sympathetic Therapeutic
Y39.-	Injection NOC
C08.4	Injection Orbit Retrobulbar
Y38.-	Injection Organ Substance Therapeutic
N32.4	Injection Penis Substance Therapeutic
C86.7	Injection Peribulbar Substance Therapeutic
K71.3	Injection Pericardium Therapeutic
H60.4	Injection Pilonidal Abscess Radiocontrast
H60.4	Injection Pilonidal Cyst Radiocontrast
H60.4	Injection Pilonidal Sinus Radiocontrast

X30.-	Injection Prophylactic NEC
X31.3	Injection Radiocontrast Intravenous NEC
X31.-	Injection Radiocontrast NEC
Y39.2	Injection Radiocontrast NOC
S53.2	Injection Scar Tissue Anaesthetic Local
X30.5	Injection Sclerosing NEC
Y09.1	Injection Sclerosing NOC
X30.3	Injection Serum Immune NEC
Y39.1	Injection Sinus Track Radiocontrast NOC
S53.-	Injection Skin NEC
V54.4	Injection Spinal Facet
X38.2	Injection Steroid NEC
C43.4	Injection Subconjunctival
X38.-	Injection Subcutaneous NEC
S51.-	Injection Subcutaneous Tissue Destructive
S50.-	Injection Subcutaneous Tissue Inert
X38.-	Injection Subcutaneous Tissue Therapeutic
C86.7	Injection Subtenons Therapeutic Substance
T74.6	Injection Tendon Blood Autologous
T74.4	Injection Tendon NEC
T74.4	Injection Tendon Sheath NEC
T74.4	Injection Tendon Therapeutic Substance NEC
Y38.1	Injection Therapeutic Continuous NOC
X30.-	Injection Therapeutic NEC
Y38.-	Injection Therapeutic NOC
X30.4	Injection Thrombin NEC
L97.7	Injection Thrombin Pseudoaneurysm
X38.1	Injection Triamcinolone
M32.3	Injection Ureteric Orifice Inert Endoscopic
Q14.-	Injection Uterine Cavity Abortifacient
Q15.3	Injection Uterine Cavity NEC
Q14.-	Injection Uterine Cavity Prostaglandin
C79.-	Injection Vitreous Body
U40.1	Inoculation Skin Intradermal Diagnostic
Q13.-	Insemination Artificial
	Insertion – see also Implantation
	Insertion – see also Injection
	Insertion – see also Introduction
L28.-	Insertion Aorta Aneurysmal Stent Endovascular
L27.-	Insertion Aorta Aneurysmal Stent Graft Endovascular
L26.7	Insertion Aorta Stent Graft Branched Transluminal NEC
L26.6	Insertion Aorta Stent Graft Fenestrated Transluminal NEC
L26.5	Insertion Aorta Stent Transluminal Percutaneous
L31.4	Insertion Artery Carotid Stent Transluminal Percutaneous
L35.3	Insertion Artery Cerebral Stent Transluminal Percutaneous
L47.4	Insertion Artery Coeliac Stent Transluminal Percutaneous
L69.5	Insertion Artery Collateral Systemic to Pulmonary Major Stent Transluminal Percutaneous
K75.-	Insertion Artery Coronary Stent & Angioplasty Balloon Transluminal Percutaneous
K75.3	Insertion Artery Coronary Stent & Angioplasty NEC
K75.1	Insertion Artery Coronary Stent Drug-eluting & Angioplasty Balloon Transluminal Percutaneous

L63.5	Insertion Artery Femoral Stent Transluminal Percutaneous
L54.4	Insertion Artery Iliac Stent Transluminal Percutaneous
L47.4	Insertion Artery Mesenteric Stent Transluminal Percutaneous
L66.7	Insertion Artery Peripheral Stent Transluminal Percutaneous
L63.5	Insertion Artery Popliteal Stent Transluminal Percutaneous
L13.6	Insertion Artery Pulmonary Stent Transluminal Percutaneous
L43.5	Insertion Artery Renal Stent Transluminal Percutaneous
L66.1	Insertion Artery Stent & Thrombolysis Transluminal Percutaneous
L66.2	Insertion Artery Stent Reconstruction Transluminal Percutaneous
L39.5	Insertion Artery Subclavian Stent Transluminal Percutaneous
L47.4	Insertion Artery Suprarenal Stent Transluminal Percutaneous
D05.1	Insertion Auricular Fixtures Prosthesis First Stage
D05.2	Insertion Auricular Fixtures Prosthesis Second Stage
M60.1	Insertion Balloon Male Continence Adjustable
R04.5	Insertion Bladder Fetus Drain Percutaneous
M55.6	Insertion Bladder Outlet Female Balloon Continence Adjustable
M55.6	Insertion Bladder Outlet Female Device Retropubic
W28.4	Insertion Bone Intramedullary Fixator & Cementing
D13.1	Insertion Bone Mastoid Prosthesis Anchored Fixture Hearing First Stage
D13.5	Insertion Bone Mastoid Prosthesis Anchored Fixture Hearing One Stage
D13.2	Insertion Bone Mastoid Prosthesis Anchored Fixture Hearing Second Stage
A10.6	Insertion Brain Neoplasm Wafer Carmustine
A09.5	Insertion Brain Neurostimulator Electrodes
C27.1	Insertion Canalicular Stent
	Insertion Cannula – see Cannulation
C77.6	Insertion Capsule Tension Ring
	Insertion Catheter – see Catheterisation
	Insertion Clip – see Clip site
H24.4	Insertion Colon Sigmoid Stent Expanding Metal Sigmoidoscope Fibreoptic
H27.4	Insertion Colon Sigmoid Stent Expanding Metal Sigmoidoscope Rigid
H21.4	Insertion Colon Stent Expanding Metal Endoscopic Fibreoptic
H31.4	Insertion Colorectal Stent Image Guided
C51.5	Insertion Cornea Contact Lens Therapeutic
A33.4	Insertion Cranial Nerve Neurostimulator Electrodes
U19.1	Insertion Electrocardiography Loop Recorder
C89.1	Insertion Eye Posterior Segment Sustained Release Device
C23.1	Insertion Eyelid Upper Weight
	Insertion Filter – see Filter site
G48.5	Insertion Gastric Balloon
G45.3	Insertion Gastrointestinal Tract Bravo Ph Capsule Endoscopic
G44.5	Insertion Gastrostomy Endoscopic Fibreoptic Percutaneous
	Insertion Implant – see Implantation
S53.-	Insertion Intradermal NEC
C64.7	Insertion Iris Hooks
W81.7	Insertion Joint Prosthesis Spacer
J15.-	Insertion Liver Blood Vessel Prosthesis Transluminal Percutaneous
V28.-	Insertion Lumbar Interspinous Process Spacer
A70.4	Insertion Nerve Peripheral Neurostimulator Electrodes
	Insertion Neurostimulator – see Neurostimulator site
G16.3	Insertion Oesophagus Bravo pH Capsule Endoscopic Fibreoptic

G19.2	Insertion Oesophagus Bravo pH Capsule Endoscopic Rigid
G15.7	Insertion Oesophagus Stent Expanding Metal Covered Endoscopic
G15.6	Insertion Oesophagus Stent Expanding Metal Endoscopic NEC
G21.5	Insertion Oesophagus Stent NEC
F14.6	Insertion Orthodontic Anchorage
F14.-	Insertion Orthodontic Appliance
F14.6	Insertion Orthodontic Screw
T12.4	Insertion Pleural Cavity Catheter Tunnelled
R04.4	Insertion Pleural Fetus Drain Percutaneous
M68.1	Insertion Prostate Stent Cystoscopic
	Insertion Prosthesis – see Prosthesis site
C29.3	Insertion Punctal Plug
H24.4	Insertion Rectum Stent Expanding Metal Sigmoidoscope Fibreoptic
H27.4	Insertion Rectum Stent Expanding Metal Sigmoidoscope Rigid
M60.1	Insertion Retropubic Male Device Continence
	Insertion Seton – see Seton site
	Insertion Shunt – see Shunt site
	Insertion Skin Expander – see Expander Skin
S53.-	Insertion Skin NEC
V18.2	Insertion Skull Distractor Internal
V18.2	Insertion Skull Spring
	Insertion Sling – see Sling site
A48.7	Insertion Spinal Cord Neurostimulator Electrodes
	Insertion Stent – see also Placement Stent
	Insertion Stent – see also Prosthesis
Y14.6	Insertion Stent Biodegradable NOC
Y14.1	Insertion Stent Expanding Metal Covered NOC
Y14.2	Insertion Stent Expanding Metal NOC
Y14.5	Insertion Stent Graft NOC
Y14.3	Insertion Stent Metal NOC
Y14.-	Insertion Stent NOC
Y14.4	Insertion Stent Plastic NOC
S52.3	Insertion Subcutaneous Tissue Beads Antibiotic
S51.-	Insertion Subcutaneous Tissue Destructive
S62.7	Insertion Subcutaneous Tissue Device Diagnostic
S52.5	Insertion Subcutaneous Tissue Hormone
S50.-	Insertion Subcutaneous Tissue Inert
S62.7	Insertion Subcutaneous Tissue Monitor Glucose
S52.5	Insertion Subcutaneous Tissue Substance Contraceptive
S62.6	Insertion Subcutaneous Tissue Substance Diagnostic
S52.-	Insertion Subcutaneous Tissue Therapeutic
	Insertion Suture – see Suture site
	Insertion System – see System
T64.-	Insertion Tendon Bone
R04.6	Insertion Tracheal Plug Fetal Percutaneous
R01.2	Insertion Tracheal Plug Fetoscopic
	Insertion Tube – see Drainage
	Insertion Tube – see Tube
M33.1	Insertion Ureter Stent Metallic Percutaneous
M33.5	Insertion Ureter Stent Percutaneous NEC

M33.2	Insertion Ureter Stent Plastic Percutaneous
M27.4	Insertion Ureter Stent Ureteroscopic
M76.6	Insertion Urethra Stent Endoscopic
P26.-	Insertion Vagina Pessary Supporting
P26.2	Insertion Vagina Ring Pessary
L97.6	Insertion Vascular Closure Device
L99.7	Insertion Vein Central Catheter Peripheral Transluminal Percutaneous
L94.3	Insertion Vein Port Subcutaneous Transluminal Percutaneous
J06.2	Insertion Vein Portal Stent Graft Intrahepatic Transjugular
J15.5	Insertion Vein Portal Stent Graft Transluminal Percutaneous
J06.1	Insertion Vein Portal Stent Intrahepatic Transjugular
J15.4	Insertion Vein Portal Stent Transluminal Percutaneous
L80.4	Insertion Vein Pulmonary Stent Transluminal Percutaneous
L99.3	Insertion Vein Stent & Thrombolysis Transluminal Percutaneous
L99.2	Insertion Vein Stent Reconstruction Transluminal Percutaneous
L94.5	Insertion Vein Stent Transluminal Percutaneous NEC
L79.3	Insertion Vena Cava Stent NEC
	Insertion Wire – see Wiring site
K53.1	Inspection Heart Valve
Y37.1	Instillation Substance Photodynamic NOC
	Instrumentation – see also Probing
V41.-	Instrumentation Spine Correction Deformity
D22.3	Insufflation Eustachian Canal
Q41.4	Insufflation Fallopian Tube
T13.1	Insufflation Pleural Cavity Talc NEC
	Interposition – see also Anastomosis
	Interposition Arthroplasty – see Arthroplasty site
L29.6	Interposition Extracranial to Intracranial High Flow
G05.-	Interposition Oesophagus NEC
L82.2	Interposition Vein Valve
	Intervention Coronary Percutaneous – see Angioplasty Artery Coronary Balloon & Insertion Stent Transluminal Percutaneous
	Intervention Coronary Percutaneous – see Angioplasty Artery Coronary Balloon Transluminal Percutaneous
N35.-	Intervention Genitalia Male Non-operative
Z99.-	Intervertebral Disc site
Z28.-	Intestine Large site
G79.-	Intestine Small Operations Endoscopic Therapeutic NEC
G82.-	Intestine Small Operations NEC
G78.-	Intestine Small Operations Open NEC
Z27.7	Intestine Small site
W71.-	Intra-articular Structure Operations NEC
X39.3	Intranasal Administration Therapeutic Subtance
	Introduction – see also Injection
	Introduction – see also Insertion
Q14.-	Introduction Amniotic Cavity Abortifacient
M53.6	Introduction Bladder Female Tape Transobturator
M64.7	Introduction Bladder Male Transobturator Sling
M49.4	Introduction Bladder Substance Therapeutic
W35.-	Introduction Bone Substance
Y35.1	Introduction Caesium Radioactive NOC
Y36.1	Introduction Gold Seeds NOC

Y36.2	Introduction Implant Therapeutic NOC
S53.-	Introduction Intradermal NEC
	Introduction Intrauterine – see Introduction Uterine Cavity
Y35.2	Introduction Iridium Wire NOC
Y36.-	Introduction Material Non-removable NOC
Y35.-	Introduction Material Radioactive Removable NOC
T48.-	Introduction Peritoneal Cavity Substance
T48.1	Introduction Peritoneal Cavity Substance Radioactive
	Introduction Pessary – see Pessary site
T13.-	Introduction Pleural Cavity Substance
Y35.3	Introduction Radium NOC
S53.-	Introduction Skin NEC
S51.-	Introduction Subcutaneous Tissue Destructive
S50.-	Introduction Subcutaneous Tissue Inert
S52.-	Introduction Subcutaneous Tissue Therapeutic
Y37.1	Introduction Substance Photodynamic NOC
Q12.1	Introduction Uterine Cavity Contraceptive Device
Q13.-	Introduction Uterine Cavity Gametes
Q15.-	Introduction Uterine Cavity Substance NEC
Q15.1	Introduction Uterine Cavity Substance Radioactive
M53.2	Introduction Vagina Bean Biethium
P26.-	Introduction Vagina Pessary Supporting Uterus Prolapse
M53.3	Introduction Vagina Tension Free Tape
	Intubation – see also Drainage
	Intubation – see also Tube site
M38.2	Intubation Bladder Suprapubic
H62.4	Intubation Bowel NEC
H30.-	Intubation Colon
G57.-	Intubation Duodenum
D22.2	Intubation Eustachian Canal
G82.-	Intubation Ileum
G78.6	Intubation Ileum Open
G82.-	Intubation Intestine Small NEC
G78.6	Intubation Intestine Small Open NEC
G67.-	Intubation Jejunum
G63.4	Intubation Jejunum Open
G21.-	Intubation Oesophagus
H46.-	Intubation Rectum
G47.-	Intubation Stomach
X56.-	Intubation Trachea
K05.-	Inversion Atrial Transposition Arteries Great
Q56.1	Investigation Fertility Female NEC
Q41.-	Investigation Fertility Female Tubal Patency
N34.1	Investigation Fertility Male NEC
Q56.1	Investigation Infertility Female NEC
Q41.-	Investigation Infertility Female Tubal Patency
N34.1	Investigation Infertility Male NEC
C59.-	Iridectomy
C59.1	Iridocyclectomy
C62.4	Iridodialysis

C60.4	Iridoplasty NEC
C62.1	Iridosclerotomy
C62.-	Iridotomy
C60.-	Iris Operations Filtering
C64.-	Iris Operations NEC
Z18.4	Iris site
D08.5	Irrigation Auditory Canal External NEC
D07.1	Irrigation Auditory Canal External Wax
M47.1	Irrigation Bladder Urethral
W33.7	Irrigation Bone NEC
H62.5	Irrigation Bowel NEC
E48.6	Irrigation Bronchus Endoscopic NEC
E50.6	Irrigation Bronchus Endoscopic Rigid
E52.1	Irrigation Bronchus NEC
E48.6	Irrigation Carina Endoscopic NEC
E50.6	Irrigation Carina Endoscopic Rigid
H30.5	Irrigation Colon
D07.1	Irrigation Ear Wax
C69.4	Irrigation Eye Anterior Chamber
W80.-	Irrigation Joint
W85.2	Irrigation Joint Knee Endoscopic
M16.1	Irrigation Kidney
C27.3	Irrigation Lacrimal Duct
E48.6	Irrigation Lung Endoscopic NEC
E50.6	Irrigation Lung Endoscopic Rigid
E12.3	Irrigation Maxillary Antrum Approach Sublabial
E13.6	Irrigation Maxillary Antrum NEC
C27.3	Irrigation Nasolacrimal Duct
Y22.3	Irrigation NOC
T46.3	Irrigation Peritoneal Cavity
E48.6	Irrigation Respiratory Tract Lower Endoscopic NEC
E50.6	Irrigation Respiratory Tract Lower Endoscopic Rigid
	Irrigation Shunt – see Shunt site
G47.3	Irrigation Stomach
E48.6	Irrigation Trachea Endoscopic NEC
E50.6	Irrigation Trachea Endoscopic Rigid
E52.1	Irrigation Trachea NEC
Z75.4	Ischium site
B08.5	Isthmectomy Thyroid

J

V19.-	Jaw Operations NEC
Z65.-	Jaw site
G58.-	Jejunectomy
G65.-	Jejunoscopy NEC
G62.-	Jejunoscopy Open
G60.-	Jejunostomy
G64.-	Jejunum Operations Endoscopic Therapeutic
G67.-	Jejunum Operations NEC
G62.-	Jejunum Operations Open Endoscopic
G63.-	Jejunum Operations Open NEC
Z27.5	Jejunum site
Z81.-	Joint Arm site NEC
Z67.1	Joint Atlanto-occipital site
Z67.2	Joint Atlantoaxial site
Z87.3	Joint Capsule site
W85.-	Joint Cavity Knee Operations Endoscopic Therapeutic
W86.-	Joint Cavity Operations Endoscopic Therapeutic NEC
Z83.-	Joint Finger site
Z86.-	Joint Foot site NEC
Z82.-	Joint Hand site NEC
Z67.-	Joint Intervertebral site
W85.-	Joint Knee Operations Endoscopic Therapeutic
Z85.-	Joint Leg Lower site
Z84.-	Joint Leg Upper site
Z87.2	Joint Ligament site
Z67.6	Joint Lumbosacral site
W77.-	Joint Operations Blocking Stabilising Joint
W86.-	Joint Operations Endoscopic Therapeutic NEC
W92.-	Joint Operations NEC
W81.-	Joint Operations Open NEC
W77.-	Joint Operations Stabilising
Z84.-	Joint Pelvis site
Z67.7	Joint Sacrococcygeal site
Z81.-	Joint Shoulder Girdle site
Z87.4	Joint site NEC
W84.-	Joint Structure Knee Operations Endoscopic Therapeutic NEC
W84.-	Joint Structure Operations Endoscopic Therapeutic NEC
W69.-	Joint Synovial Membrane Operations Open
Z85.-	Joint Tarsus site NEC
V21.-	Joint Temporomandibular Operations NEC
Z65.2	Joint Temporomandibular site
W79.-	Joint Toe Operations Soft Tissue
Z82.-	Joint Wrist site
Z40.4	Jugular Body site

K

C45.1	Keratectomy Laser
C44.4	Keratectomy Photorefractive
C45.1	Keratectomy Superficial
C44.2	Keratomileusis Laser in Situ
C44.5	Keratomileusis Subepithelial Laser
C44.3	Keratoplasty Endothelial
C46.5	Keratoplasty Lamellar Deep
C46.2	Keratoplasty Lamellar NEC
C46.3	Keratoplasty Penetrating
C44.1	Keratoplasty Prosthetic Hydrogel
C46.1	Keratoplasty Refractive
C49.3	Keratotomy Radial
M09.-	Kidney Calculus Operations Endoscopic Therapeutic
M10.-	Kidney Operations Endoscopic Therapeutic NEC
M16.-	Kidney Operations NEC
M15.-	Kidney Operations Nephrostomy Tube Track
M08.-	Kidney Operations Open NEC
M08.-	Kidney Pelvis Operations Open NEC
Z41.1	Kidney site
O13.2	Knee site NEC (Z)
V44.5	Kyphoplasty Spine Fracture Balloon

L

D26.-	Labyrinthectomy
C29.-	Lacrimal Apparatus Operations NEC
Z16.7	Lacrimal Apparatus site
C24.-	Lacrimal Gland Operations
Z16.5	Lacrimal Gland site
C26.-	Lacrimal Sac Operations NEC
Z16.6	Lacrimal Sac site
	Laminectomy – see also Excision Disc Intervertebral
V49.-	Laminectomy Exploratory
Y48.-	Laminectomy Spine Approach
V22.7	Laminoplasty Spine Cervical NEC
V23.7	Laminoplasty Spine Cervical Revisional
	Laparoscopic – refer to Index Introduction
Y75.-	Laparoscopic Approach NEC
T43.-	Laparoscopy
Q39.-	Laparoscopy Fallopian Tube
T43.-	Laparoscopy Gynaecological
Q50.-	Laparoscopy Ovary
Y50.2	Laparotomy Approach NEC
T30.-	Laparotomy Exploratory
S58.-	Larvae Therapy
E29.-	Laryngectomy Open
E35.6	Laryngectomy Partial Endoscopic
E29.5	Laryngofissure & Chordectomy Vocal Chord
E36.-	Laryngoscopy
E31.2	Laryngotracheoplasty NEC
E33.3	Larynx Cartilage Operations NEC
E34.-	Larynx Operations Endoscopic Microtherapeutic
E35.-	Larynx Operations Endoscopic Therapeutic NEC
E38.-	Larynx Operations NEC
E33.-	Larynx Operations Open NEC
Z24.2	Larynx site
Y08.-	Laser NOC
Y71.-	Late Operations NOC
Z94.-	Laterality Operations
	Lavage – see also Irrigation
E49.-	Lavage Respiratory Tract Lower Endoscopic Fibreoptic
E49.-	Lavage Respiratory Tract Lower Endoscopic NEC
	Laying Open – see Opening
S59.-	Leech Therapy

S59.2	Leech Therapy Skin
S59.1	Leech Therapy Skin Head
S59.1	Leech Therapy Skin Neck
Z94.3	Left Sided Operations
Z90.-	Leg Region site NEC
O13.-	Leg Region site Other NEC (Z)
W17.-	Lengthening Bone
C35.2	Lengthening Eye Muscle Slide
T70.5	Lengthening Muscle
C35.2	Lengthening Muscle Eye Slide
T70.5	Lengthening Tendon
C77.-	Lens Operations NEC
Z19.1	Lens site
C74.3	Lensectomy Mechanical
C74.3	Lensectomy Pars Plana
X32.7	Leucopheresis
A10.1	Leucotomy NEC
A03.1	Leucotomy Stereotactic
V55.-	Levels Spine
	Lift – see also Elevation
S01.4	Lift Brow
S03.1	Lift Buttock
S01.-	Lift Face
S03.2	Lift Thigh
Q52.-	Ligament Broad Uterus Operations NEC
W76.-	Ligament Operations NEC
Z87.2	Ligament site
Q54.-	Ligament Uterus Operations NEC
	Ligation – see also Occlusion
L75.2	Ligation Arteriovenous Fistula Acquired
L75.1	Ligation Arteriovenous Malformation Congenital
L38.2	Ligation Artery Axillary
L38.2	Ligation Artery Brachial
L30.2	Ligation Artery Carotid
L33.3	Ligation Artery Cerebral Aneurysmal
L33.3	Ligation Artery Circle Willis Aneurysmal
L46.3	Ligation Artery Coeliac
E12.1	Ligation Artery Maxillary Approach Sublabial
L46.3	Ligation Artery Mesenteric
L70.3	Ligation Artery NEC
E05.2	Ligation Artery Nose Internal
L62.3	Ligation Artery Popliteal Aneurysmal
L12.6	Ligation Artery Pulmonary
L42.3	Ligation Artery Renal
L38.2	Ligation Artery Subclavian
L46.3	Ligation Artery Suprarenal
L38.2	Ligation Artery Vertebral
L02.2	Ligation Ductus Arteriosus Patent
Q27.1	Ligation Fallopian Tube Bilateral Open
Q28.-	Ligation Fallopian Tube Open NEC

G43.7	Ligation Gastrointestinal Tract Upper Rubber Band Endoscopic Fibreoptic
H52.4	Ligation Haemorrhoid
L85.-	Ligation Leg Vein Varicose
E57.2	Ligation Lung Bulla
T89.3	Ligation Lymphatic Duct
Y07.1	Ligation NOC
E05.2	Ligation Nose Internal Artery
G10.4	Ligation Oesophagus Varices Local
G43.7	Ligation Oesophagus Varices Rubber Band Endoscopic Fibreoptic
F52.1	Ligation Parotid Duct
T19.3	Ligation Patent Processus Vaginalis
F52.-	Ligation Salivary Duct
K55.1	Ligation Sinus Valsalva
F52.2	Ligation Submandibular Duct
N19.1	Ligation Varicocele
N17.2	Ligation Vas Deferens NEC
L93.3	Ligation Vein NEC
L83.2	Ligation Vein Perforating Leg Subfascial Open
	Ligature – see Ligation
	Ligature Removal – see Removal from site Ligature
S12.-	Light Therapy Skin Ultraviolet
L91.3	Linogram Venous Catheter Central
F06.-	Lip Mucosa Operations NEC
F06.-	Lip Operations NEC
Z25.1	Lip site
F06.-	Lip Skin Operations NEC
Z25.1	Lip Skin site
S02.2	Lipectomy Abdominal
S03.3	Lipectomy NEC
S01.3	Lipectomy Submental
B37.5	Lipofilling Breast
Y39.4	Lipofilling Organ Injection
S62.-	Liposuction Subcutaneous Tissue
M44.1	Lithopaxy Endoscopic
	Lithotripsy – see also Fragmentation
N27.4	Lithotripsy Penis Lesion Extracorporeal Shockwave
T74.5	Lithotripsy Tendon Calculus Extracorporeal Shockwave
J11.-	Liver Blood Vessel Operations Transjugular Intrahepatic
J06.-	Liver Blood Vessel Operations Transjugular Intrahepatic Other
J10.-	Liver Blood Vessel Operations Transluminal
J77.-	Liver Blood Vessel Operations Transluminal Other
X43.-	Liver Failure Compensation
J08.-	Liver Operations Endoscopic Therapeutic
J08.-	Liver Operations Laparoscope
J16.-	Liver Operations NEC
J07.-	Liver Operations Open NEC
J13.-	Liver Operations Percutaneous Diagnostic
J12.-	Liver Operations Percutaneous Therapeutic NEC
J08.-	Liver Operations Peritonoscope
Z30.1	Liver site

A01.-	Lobectomy Brain
E54.-	Lobectomy Lung
B08.4	Lobectomy Thyroid NEC
Z10.-	Lumbar Plexus site
B28.3	Lumpectomy Breast
Z72.3	Lunate site
E48.-	Lung Operations Endoscopic NEC
E50.-	Lung Operations Endoscopic Rigid
E59.-	Lung Operations NEC
E57.-	Lung Operations Open NEC
Z24.6	Lung site
T91.-	Lymph Node Operations Sentinel
O14.2	Lymph Node Sentinal (Z)
Z61.-	Lymph Node site
O14.-	Lymph Node site Other (Z)
T90.-	Lymphangiography
T89.-	Lymphatic Duct Operations
Z62.2	Lymphatic Duct site
T92.-	Lymphatic Tissue Operations NEC
Z62.3	Lymphatic Tissue site

M

H57.2	Maintenance Anal Sphincter Artificial NEC
	Maintenance Pack – see Packing
	Maintenance Prosthesis – see Prosthesis site
	Maintenance Shunt – see Shunt site
H57.6	Maintenance Sphincter Dynamic Graciloplasty
Y15.1	Maintenance Stent NOC
	Maintenance System – see System
Z78.4	Malleolus Lateral site
Z77.3	Malleolus Medial site
B34.-	Mammary Duct Operations
U18.3	Mammography
B31.-	Mammoplasty
V19.-	Mandible Operations NEC
Z65.1	Mandible site
V14.-	Mandibulectomy
	Manipulation – see also Remanipulation
W26.-	Manipulation Bone Fracture
W25.-	Manipulation Bone Fracture & Fixation External
V09.2	Manipulation Bone Nose Fracture
H17.-	Manipulation Caecum Intra-abdominal
H17.-	Manipulation Colon Intra-abdominal
Y42.1	Manipulation External NOC
G76.-	Manipulation Ileum Intra-abdominal
G76.-	Manipulation Intestine Small Intra-abdominal NEC
V19.5	Manipulation Jaw NEC
W66.-	Manipulation Joint Dislocation Fracture
W66.-	Manipulation Joint Dislocation NEC
W91.-	Manipulation Joint NEC
W91.3	Manipulation Joint Prosthetic NEC
W91.1	Manipulation Joint Traction NEC
V19.5	Manipulation Mandible NEC
Y42.-	Manipulation NOC
H44.-	Manipulation Rectum
V50.-	Manipulation Spine
Q20.3	Manipulation Uterus Manual
L72.2	Manometry Arterial NEC
M49.8	Manometry Bladder
A11.3	Manometry Brain Tissue
A20.3	Manometry Brain Ventricle
H30.2	Manometry Colon

H30.2	Manometry Intestine NEC
T83.5	Manometry Muscle Compartment Catheter
Y44.2	Manometry NOC
G21.-	Manometry Oesophagus
H46.3	Manometry Rectum
A55.3	Manometry Spinal
G47.-	Manometry Stomach
J11.7	Manometry Vein Hepatic Intrahepatic Transjugular
L95.2	Manometry Vein NEC
J11.6	Manometry Vein Portal Intrahepatic Transjugular
	Mapping – see Study
A11.4	Mapping Cortical
	Marsupialisation – see also Deroofing
	Marsupialisation – see also Excision
P03.2	Marsupialisation Bartholin Gland
C29.4	Marsupialisation Canaliculus
F18.2	Marsupialisation Jaw Lesion Dental
J02.5	Marsupialisation Liver Lesion
Y06.1	Marsupialisation NOC
Q43.3	Marsupialisation Ovary Lesion
J70.2	Marsupialisation Spleen Lesion
P17.3	Marsupialisation Vagina Lesion
X61.3	Massage Body
K55.2	Massage Heart Chest Open
M70.5	Massage Prostate
H44.5	Massage Rectum
B27.-	Mastectomy
D12.-	Mastoid Operations NEC
Z20.3	Mastoid site
D10.-	Mastoidectomy
B31.3	Mastopexy
Z64.4	Maxilla site
E12.-	Maxillary Antrum Operations Approach Sublabial
E13.-	Maxillary Antrum Operations NEC
Z23.1	Maxillary Antrum site
V06.-	Maxillectomy
	Measurement – see Manometry
	Measurement – see Study
D03.4	Meatoplasty Ear External
M81.2	Meatoplasty Urethra
M32.2	Meatotomy Ureteric Orifice Endoscopic
M81.3	Meatotomy Urethral Orifice External
E35.7	Medialisation Vocal Cord Endoscopic
E33.6	Medialisation Vocal Cord Using Biological Implant
E33.5	Medialisation Vocal Cord Using Implant
E63.-	Mediastinoscopy
E63.-	Mediastinoscopy Cervical
E61.4	Mediastinotomy NEC
E62.-	Mediastinum Operations Endoscopic Therapeutic
E61.-	Mediastinum Operations Open

Z24.7	Mediastinum site
C80.-	Membrane Retina Operations
C73.1	Membranectomy Lens
W82.-	Meniscectomy Endoscopic
V21.1	Meniscectomy Joint Temporomandibular
W70.-	Meniscectomy NEC
T38.-	Mesentery Colon Operations
T37.-	Mesentery Intestine Small Operations
Z53.6	Mesentery site
Q17.5	Metroplasty Endoscopic
Q09.5	Metroplasty Open
V29.6	Microdiscectomy Disc Intervertebral Cervical NEC
V30.6	Microdiscectomy Disc Intervertebral Cervical Revisional
V33.7	Microdiscectomy Disc Intervertebral Lumbar NEC
V34.7	Microdiscectomy Disc Intervertebral Lumbar Revisional
B34.4	Microdochotomy
W84.5	Microfracture Bone Cartilage Articular Repair
E37.-	Microlaryngoscopy
	Microwave – see Destruction
K38.3	Mitral Subvalvar Apparatus Operations
H62.2	Mobilisation Bowel NEC
	Monitoring – see also Establishing
U19.6	Monitoring Cardiomemo Electrocardiographic
Y73.6	Monitoring Intraoperative Fluid
Y73.6	Monitoring Oesophageal Doppler
	Monitoring Pressure – see Manometry
W83.7	Mosaicplasty Endoscopic
F42.-	Mouth Operations NEC
F40.5	Mouth Removal Suture NEC
Z25.-	Mouth site
X61.4	Movement Therapy
	Muscle – see also site Muscle
Z60.3	Muscle Abdominal Wall Anterior site
Z54.-	Muscle Arm Upper site
Z60.4	Muscle Back site
Z60.5	Muscle Chest site
E28.-	Muscle Cricopharyngeus Operations
C31.-	Muscle Eye Operations Combined
C37.-	Muscle Eye Operations NEC
Z17.-	Muscle Eye site NEC
Z60.1	Muscle Face site
Z59.-	Muscle Foot site
Z55.-	Muscle Forearm site
Z56.-	Muscle Hand site
Z57.-	Muscle Hip site
Z58.-	Muscle Leg Lower site
Z60.2	Muscle Neck site
T83.-	Muscle Operations NEC
Z54.-	Muscle Shoulder site
Z60.-	Muscle site NEC

Z57.-	Muscle Thigh site
Z60.5	Muscle Thorax site
Z87.-	Musculoskeletal System site NEC
K24.6	Myectomy Ventricular Outflow Tract
A55.1	Myelography Lumbar
A55.2	Myelography Spinal NEC
A45.3	Myelotomy Spinal Cord
A45.3	Myelotomy Spinal Tract
Q09.2	Myomectomy Open
E28.1	Myotomy Cricopharyngeal
M41.6	Myotomy Detrusor
T83.2	Myotomy NEC
K24.7	Myotomy Ventricular Outflow Tract
D14.-	Myringoplasty
D15.-	Myringotomy

N

S66.-	Nail Bed Operations NEC
Z51.1	Nail Bed site
S70.-	Nail Operations NEC
Z51.-	Nail site
E64.-	Nasal Cavity Operations Endoscopic Therapeutic
E17.-	Nasal Sinus Operations NEC
Z23.-	Nasal Sinus site
E65.-	Nasendoscopy
C27.-	Nasolacrimal Duct Operations
E21.-	Nasopharyngoplasty
E25.-	Nasopharyngoscopy
E24.-	Nasopharynx Operations Endoscopic Therapeutic
E27.-	Nasopharynx Operations NEC
E23.-	Nasopharynx Operations Open NEC
Z22.6	Nasopharynx site
Z79.3	Navicular site
E89.3	Nebuliser NEC
J57.6	Necrosectomy Pancreatic
C65.1	Needling Bleb Following Glaucoma Surgery
C71.1	Needling Lens Cataract
A47.1	Needling Spinal Cord Cervical Substantia Gelatinosa
M02.-	Nephrectomy NEC
M03.-	Nephrectomy Partial NEC
M06.1	Nephrolithotomy
M16.4	Nephrolithotomy Percutaneous NEC
M05.3	Nephropexy
M11.-	Nephroscopy
M15.1	Nephrostomography
	Nephrostomy – see also Drainage Kidney
M06.-	Nephrostomy
M13.6	Nephrostomy Tube Insertion Percutaneous
M02.-	Nephroureterectomy
Z09.-	Nerve Arm Peripheral site
Y82.1	Nerve Block Anaesthetic
	Nerve Block Destructive – see Denervation site
	Nerve Block Destructive – see Destruction Nerve
Y82.1	Nerve Block NEC
Z09.1	Nerve Circumflex site
A84.3	Nerve Conduction Studies
A36.-	Nerve Cranial Operations NEC

Z04.-	Nerve Cranial site NEC
Z03.-	Nerve Cranial Upper site
Z10.3	Nerve Cutaneous Lateral Thigh site
Z09.-	Nerve Digital Finger site
Z12.5	Nerve Digital Toe site
Z10.1	Nerve Femoral site
Z09.-	Nerve Finger site
Z10.5	Nerve Iliohypogastric site
Z10.4	Nerve Ilioinguinal site
Z09.6	Nerve Interosseous Anterior site
Z09.5	Nerve Interosseous Posterior site
Z12.6	Nerve Leg Peripheral site NEC
Z09.2	Nerve Median site
Z10.2	Nerve Obturator site
Z09.-	Nerve Peripheral Arm site
Z12.6	Nerve Peripheral Leg site NEC
A73.-	Nerve Peripheral Operations NEC
Z12.-	Nerve Peripheral site
Z12.4	Nerve Plantar site
Z12.1	Nerve Popliteal site
Z09.3	Nerve Radial site
A57.-	Nerve Root Spinal Ganglion Operations
A57.-	Nerve Root Spinal Operations
Z07.-	Nerve Root Spinal site
Z11.2	Nerve Sacral site
Z11.1	Nerve Sciatic site
Z12.-	Nerve site NEC
Z12.3	Nerve Sural site
A81.-	Nerve Sympathetic Operations NEC
Z12.7	Nerve Sympathetic site
Z10.3	Nerve Thigh Cutaneous Lateral site
Z12.2	Nerve Tibial Posterior site
Z12.5	Nerve Toe Digital site
Z09.4	Nerve Ulna site
D24.4	Neurectomy Cochlea
A59.-	Neurectomy NEC
E13.7	Neurectomy Nerve Vidian NEC
E12.4	Neurectomy Nerve Vidian Transantral Approach Sublabial
D26.4	Neurectomy Vestibular Apparatus
	Neurolysis – see also Release Nerve Entrapment
A31.-	Neurolysis Nerve Cranial Intracranial Stereotactic
A68.-	Neurolysis Nerve Peripheral NEC
A69.-	Neurolysis Nerve Peripheral Revision
A84.-	Neurophysiological Operations
	Neurostimulation – see Neurostimulator
A09.-	Neurostimulator Brain
A33.-	Neurostimulator Nerve Cranial
A70.-	Neurostimulator Nerve Peripheral
A48.-	Neurostimulator Spinal Cord
A36.4	Neurotomy Optic Radial (ii)

B35.-	Nipple Operations
B35.4	Nipple Operations Plastic
Z15.6	Nipple site
B35.-	Nipple Skin Operations
Z15.6	Nipple Skin site
Y90.-	Non-operations NEC
E09.-	Nose External Operations
Z22.-	Nose External site
E09.-	Nose External Skin Operations
Z22.-	Nose External Skin site
E08.-	Nose Internal Operations NEC
E10.-	Nose Operations NEC
E02.-	Nose Operations Plastic
E07.-	Nose Operations Plastic Other
E03.-	Nose Septum Operations
E16.-	Nose Sinuses Endoscopic Examination Diagnostic
Z22.-	Nose site NEC
E04.-	Nose Turbinate Operations
U23.-	Nuclear Medicine Haematological Tests

O

L33.4	Obliteration Artery Cerebral Aneurysmal NEC
L33.4	Obliteration Artery Circle Willis Aneurysmal NEC
Y07.-	Obliteration Cavity NOC
Y07.4	Obliteration Diverticulum NOC
Y07.3	Obliteration Fistula NOC
D12.1	Obliteration Mastoid
Y07.3	Obliteration Sinus Track NOC
P18.-	Obliteration Vagina NEC
R34.-	Obstetric Operations NEC
	Occlusion – see also Ligation
L08.7	Occlusion Artery Anastomosis Subclavian Pulmonary Transluminal Percutaneous
L66.4	Occlusion Artery Balloon Test Transluminal Percutaneous
L69.1	Occlusion Artery Collateral Systemic to Pulmonary Major
K78.1	Occlusion Artery Mammary Left Internal Side Branch Transluminal Percutaneous
L07.5	Occlusion Artery Shunt Subclavian Pulmonary Transluminal Percutaneous
L66.3	Occlusion Artery Transluminal Percutaneous
K22.3	Occlusion Atrial Appendage Left NEC
K62.5	Occlusion Atrial Appendage Left Transluminal Percutaneous
H31.-	Occlusion Colorectal Fistula Image Guided
H31.1	Occlusion Colorectal Fistula Percutaneous Image Guided
H31.2	Occlusion Colorectal Fistula Transluminal Image Guided
L03.1	Occlusion Ductus Arteriosus Patent Prosthetic Transluminal Percutaneous
Q35.-	Occlusion Fallopian Tube Bilateral Access Minimal
Q35.-	Occlusion Fallopian Tube Bilateral Endoscopic NEC
Q27.-	Occlusion Fallopian Tube Bilateral Open
Q36.-	Occlusion Fallopian Tube Endoscopic NEC
Q28.-	Occlusion Fallopian Tube Open NEC
C29.3	Occlusion Lacrimal Punctum
Y07.5	Occlusion NOC
Y44.3	Occlusion Organ Temporary
L99.6	Occlusion Vein Balloon Test Transluminal Percutaneous
L99.5	Occlusion Vein Transluminal Percutaneous
Y44.3	Occlusion Vessel Temporary
G03.-	Oesophagectomy NEC
G03.-	Oesophagectomy Partial
G02.-	Oesophagectomy Total
G01.-	Oesophagogastrectomy
G09.2	Oesophagomyotomy NEC
G16.-	Oesophagoscopy Fibreoptic
G16.-	Oesophagoscopy NEC

G08.-	Oesophagostomy
Y51.1	Oesophagostomy Approach
G15.-	Oesophagus Operations Endoscopic Fibreoptic Therapeutic NEC
G15.-	Oesophagus Operations Endoscopic Therapeutic NEC
G21.-	Oesophagus Operations NEC
G13.-	Oesophagus Operations Open NEC
Z27.1	Oesophagus site
G10.-	Oesophagus Varices Operations Open
T36.1	Omentectomy
T36.-	Omentum Operations
Z53.5	Omentum site
Q48.-	Oocyte Recovery
Q48.-	Oocyte Recovery Access Minimal
Q22.3	Oophorectomy Bilateral NEC
Q24.3	Oophorectomy NEC
Q23.-	Oophorectomy Unilateral NEC
	Opening – see also Exteriorisation
	Opening – see also Reopening
T30.-	Opening Abdomen
T30.-	Opening Abdominal Wall
H55.-	Opening Anal Fistula
Y52.-	Opening Artificial Approach NEC
T03.-	Opening Chest
T03.-	Opening Chest Wall
V01.3	Opening Cranial Suture
V03.-	Opening Cranium
G75.-	Opening Ileum Artificial Attention
G74.-	Opening Ileum Artificial Creation
G75.-	Opening Intestine Small Artificial Attention NEC
G74.-	Opening Intestine Small Artificial Creation NEC
G60.-	Opening Jejunum Artificial
G08.-	Opening Oesophagus Artificial
T30.-	Opening Peritoneal Cavity
T30.-	Opening Peritoneum
H60.2	Opening Pilonidal Abscess
H60.2	Opening Pilonidal Cyst
H60.2	Opening Pilonidal Sinus
T03.-	Opening Pleura
T03.-	Opening Pleural Cavity
S47.-	Opening Skin
G34.-	Opening Stomach Artificial NEC
S47.-	Opening Subcutaneous Tissue
	Operations Abandoned – refer to Tabular List Introduction
H57.-	Operations Anal Sphincter Incontinence Control Other
L69.-	Operations Arteries Collateral Systemic to Pulmonary Major
K78.-	Operations Artery Mammary Internal Side Branch Transluminal
L66.-	Operations Artery Therapeutic Transluminal Other
Z94.1	Operations Bilateral
Y70.-	Operations Early NOC
Y70.1	Operations Emergency NOC

C89.-	Operations Eye Posterior Segment
Y73.-	Operations Facilitating NOC
	Operations Failed – refer to Tabular List Introduction
Y70.2	Operations Immediate NOC
	Operations Incomplete – refer to Tabular List Introduction
Y71.-	Operations Late NOC
Z94.-	Operations Laterality
Z94.3	Operations Left Sided
Y44.-	Operations Methods NOC
Y70.4	Operations Primary NOC
	Operations Radical – refer to Tabular List Introduction
Y71.3	Operations Revisional NOC
Y71.6	Operations Revisional Second NOC
Y71.7	Operations Revisional Third or Greater NOC
Z94.2	Operations Right Sided
Y71.2	Operations Secondary NOC
Y70.3	Operations Staged First NOC
Y71.1	Operations Staged Subsequent NOC
Y70.5	Operations Temporary
	Operations Unfinished – refer to Tabular List Introduction
Z94.4	Operations Unilateral
C87.5	Ophthalmoscopy Retina Scanning Laser
X39.1	Oral Administration Therapeutic Substance
F11.-	Oral Surgery Preprosthetic
C08.-	Orbit Operations NEC
Z16.1	Orbit site
C06.-	Orbitotomy
N05.-	Orchidectomy Bilateral
N06.6	Orchidectomy Inguinal & Excision Cord Spermatic NEC
N05.3	Orchidectomy Inguinal Bilateral
N05.3	Orchidectomy Inguinal Bilateral & Excision Cord Spermatic
N06.6	Orchidectomy Inguinal NEC
N06.-	Orchidectomy NEC
N08.-	Orchidopexy Bilateral
N09.-	Orchidopexy NEC
X55.-	Organ Unspecified Operations NEC
F14.-	Orthodontic Appliance
F15.-	Orthodontic Appliance Other
F14.-	Orthodontic Operations
F15.-	Orthodontic Operations Other
Z79.2	Os Calcis site
W06.-	Ostectomy NEC
W11.1	Osteoclasis Closed
W10.-	Osteoclasis NEC
W10.-	Osteoclasis Open
E16.1	Osteoplasty Frontal Sinus
V10.6	Osteotomy Bone Face & Translocation Orbit
V10.-	Osteotomy Bone Face NEC
V10.7	Osteotomy Bone Face Subcranial U
W15.7	Osteotomy Bone Foot & Fixation

V10.6	Osteotomy Box Orbit
W13.3	Osteotomy Cuneiform NEC
W13.4	Osteotomy Derotation & Relocation
W14.-	Osteotomy Diaphyseal
W13.2	Osteotomy Displacement
V16.-	Osteotomy Jaw NEC
V16.1	Osteotomy Mandible & Advancement
V16.2	Osteotomy Mandible & Retrusion
V16.3	Osteotomy Mandible Dentoalveolar Level
V16.-	Osteotomy Mandible NEC
V10.5	Osteotomy Maxilla Dentoalveolar Level
V10.-	Osteotomy Maxilla NEC
W15.-	Osteotomy Metatarsal
W03.2	Osteotomy Metatarsal Multiple
W03.6	Osteotomy Metatarsals Multiple & Fixation
W16.-	Osteotomy Multiple NEC
W16.-	Osteotomy NEC
X25.1	Osteotomy Os Calcis Body
X22.-	Osteotomy Pelvis Correction Hip Deformity Congenital
W12.-	Osteotomy Periarticular Angulation
W13.1	Osteotomy Periarticular Rotation
W77.5	Osteotomy Periarticular Stabilising Joint
W15.6	Osteotomy Phalanx Proximal Cuneiform & Resection First Metatarsal Head
W15.6	Osteotomy Phalanx Proximal Wedge & Resection First Metatarsal Head
W13.4	Osteotomy Relocation & Derotation
V54.3	Osteotomy Spine NEC
W15.-	Osteotomy Tarsal
W13.3	Osteotomy Wedge NEC
E04.7	Outfracture Nose Turbinate Surgical
Q45.2	Ovariopexy
Q49.-	Ovary Operations Endoscopic Therapeutic
Q47.-	Ovary Operations Open NEC
Q51.-	Ovary Operations Other
Z46.3	Ovary site
M43.3	Overdistension Bladder Endoscopic NEC
	Oversewing – see Closure
E91.1	Oximetry Assessment
E91.2	Oximetry Continuous
E91.3	Oximetry Overnight
E91.-	Oximetry Testing
E87.3	Oxygen Ambulatory
E87.1	Oxygen Support Home
X52.-	Oxygen Therapy
E87.2	Oxygen Therapy Long Term
X58.1	Oxygenation Extracorporeal Membrane

P

J04.3	Packing Liver Laceration
D12.-	Packing Mastoid Cavity
E06.-	Packing Nose Cavity
F16.3	Packing Tooth Socket
F32.-	Palate Operations NEC
Z25.6	Palate site
J68.-	Pancreas Operations NEC
J65.-	Pancreas Operations Open NEC
J67.-	Pancreas Operations Percutaneous Diagnostic
J66.-	Pancreas Operations Percutaneous Therapeutic
Z31.1	Pancreas site
J57.-	Pancreatectomy NEC
J55.-	Pancreatectomy Total
J42.-	Pancreatic Duct Operations Endoscopic Therapeutic Retrograde
J60.-	Pancreatic Duct Operations Open NEC
Z31.2	Pancreatic Duct site
J56.-	Pancreaticoduodenectomy
J67.2	Pancreatography & Puncture Pancreatic Duct Percutaneous
J45.-	Pancreatography Endoscopic Retrograde
J63.-	Pancreatography Open
H04.-	Panproctocolectomy & Anastomosis Ileum Anus
H04.1	Panproctocolectomy & Ileostomy
Q55.-	Papanicolau Smear
J39.-	Papilla Vater Operations Endoscopic Therapeutic NEC
J36.-	Papilla Vater Operations NEC
Z30.6	Papilla Vater site
K38.1	Papillary Muscle Operations
T46.1	Paracentesis Abdominis Ascites
T12.2	Paracentesis Chest
C69.2	Paracentesis Eye Anterior Chamber
B16.-	Parathyroid Operations NEC
Z13.5	Parathyroid site
B14.-	Parathyroidectomy
F58.1	Parotid Duct Operations NEC
F53.1	Parotid Duct Operations Open NEC
Z26.5	Parotid Duct site
Z26.1	Parotid Gland site
F44.-	Parotidectomy
G30.2	Partitioning Stomach NEC
G30.3	Partitioning Stomach Using Band

G30.4	Partitioning Stomach Using Staples
A52.3	Patch Epidural Blood
U27.-	Patch Test Skin
Z78.7	Patella site
Q41.5	Patency Fallopian Tube NEC
C80.1	Peel Epiretinal Fibroglial Membrane
C80.1	Peel Epiretinal Membrane
C80.2	Peel Retina Internal Limiting Membrane
Z75.-	Pelvis site
O16.1	Pelvis site NEC (Z)
N32.6	Penis Operations Erectile Dysfunction NEC
N32.-	Penis Operations NEC
N28.-	Penis Operations Plastic
Z42.7	Penis site
N32.-	Penis Skin Operations NEC
N28.-	Penis Skin Operations Plastic
Z42.7	Penis Skin site
K35.6	Perforation Valve Pulmonary Transluminal Percutaneous & Dilation
L97.3	Perfusion Limb Isolated
J07.2	Perfusion Liver Cannula Insertion Open
J16.1	Perfusion Liver Localised
H55.-	Perianal Region Operations NEC
Z29.3	Perianal Tissue site
K68.2	Pericardiocentesis NEC
K77.1	Pericardiocentesis Transluminal
K71.-	Pericardium Operations NEC
Z33.5	Pericardium site
P13.3	Perineoplasty Female
P13.2	Perineorrhaphy Female
P13.5	Perineotomy Female NEC
P13.-	Perineum Female Operations NEC
Z44.4	Perineum Female site
N24.-	Perineum Male Operations
Z43.6	Perineum Male site
P13.-	Perineum Skin Female Operations NEC
Z44.4	Perineum Skin Female site
N24.-	Perineum Skin Male Operations
Z43.6	Perineum Skin Male site
C41.1	Peritomy
T48.-	Peritoneal Cavity Introduction Substance
T42.-	Peritoneal Cavity Operations Endoscopic Therapeutic
T48.-	Peritoneal Cavity Operations NEC
T41.-	Peritoneal Cavity Operations Open NEC
Z53.4	Peritoneal Cavity site
T43.-	Peritoneoscopy
T42.-	Peritoneum Operations Endoscopic Therapeutic
T48.-	Peritoneum Operations NEC
T41.-	Peritoneum Operations Open NEC
T39.-	Peritoneum Posterior Operations
Z53.3	Peritoneum site

F36.-	Peritonsillar Region Operations
Z25.7	Peritonsillar Region site
P13.6	Periurethral Tissue Female Operations NEC
Q14.6	Pessary Abortifacient NEC
Q14.5	Pessary Prostaglandin
P26.-	Pessary Vagina Supporting
C71.2	Phacoemulsification Lens
C71.2	Phacolensectomy
E23.2	Pharyngeal Pouch Operations
E24.3	Pharyngeal Pouch Operations Endoscopic Therapeutic
E19.-	Pharyngectomy
E21.-	Pharyngoplasty
E25.-	Pharyngoscopy
E24.-	Pharynx Operations Endoscopic Therapeutic
E27.-	Pharynx Operations NEC
E23.-	Pharynx Operations Open NEC
Z24.1	Pharynx site
S64.2	Phenolisation Nail Bed
L87.7	Phlebectomy Transilluminated Powered Leg Vein Varicose
S12.-	Photochemotherapy Skin
S12.-	Photochemotherapy Skin Combined & Light Therapy Ultraviolet
C66.4	Photocoagulation Ciliary Body Laser
C81.-	Photocoagulation Retina Detachment
C82.6	Photocoagulation Retina Lesion Laser NEC
C82.5	Photocoagulation Retina Lesion Laser Panretinal
C82.-	Photocoagulation Retina NEC
S09.-	Photocoagulation Skin Lesion Infrared
	Photodestruction – see also Destruction
S09.-	Photodestruction Skin Lesion NEC
S09.-	Photodestruction Subcutaneous Tissue Lesion NEC
J41.4	Photodynamic Therapy Bile Duct Lesion Laser Endoscopic Retrograde
J48.4	Photodynamic Therapy Bile Duct Lesion Percutaneous
G42.2	Photodynamic Therapy Gastrointestinal Tract Upper Lesion Endo. Fibreoptic
G42.2	Photodynamic Therapy Gastrointestinal Tract Upper Lesion Endoscopic NEC
Y13.6	Photodynamic Therapy NOC
G14.7	Photodynamic Therapy Oesophagus Lesion Endoscopic Fibreoptic
E48.7	Photodynamic Therapy Respiratory Tract Lower Lesion Endoscopic Fibreoptic
S07.-	Photodynamic Therapy Skin
C88.2	Photodynamic Therapy Subretina Lesion
F42.4	Photography Mouth
U27.7	Photopatch Testing Skin
U28.-	Phototesting Skin
S12.-	Phototherapy Skin
H60.-	Pilonidal Abscess Operations NEC
H60.-	Pilonidal Cyst Operations NEC
H60.-	Pilonidal Sinus Operations NEC
B06.-	Pineal Operations
Z14.2	Pineal site
D03.3	Pinnaplasty
W19.1	Pinning & Plating Femur Neck Fracture NEC

W24.1	Pinning Femur Neck Fracture NEC
B04.-	Pituitary Operations NEC
Z14.1	Pituitary site
B04.5	Pituitary Stalk Operations
H57.1	Placement Anal Sphincter Artificial NEC
J40.-	Placement Bile Duct Stent Endoscopic Retrograde
C51.5	Placement Cornea Therapeutic Contact Lens
A11.1	Placement Depth Electrodes Electroencephalography
D05.5	Placement Ear External Hearing Implant
D20.4	Placement Ear Middle Hearing Implant
Q35.4	Placement Intrafallopian Implant Bilateral Endoscopic
Q36.2	Placement Intrafallopian Implant Solitary Endoscopic
	Placement Prosthesis – see Prosthesis site
H57.5	Placement Sphincter Dynamic Graciloplasty
L89.-	Placement Stent Coated Endovascular
L89.-	Placement Stent Drug-eluting Endovascular
L76.-	Placement Stent Endovascular
O20.1	Placement Stent Graft Branched One Endovascular (L)
O20.-	Placement Stent Graft Endovascular (L)
O20.2	Placement Stent Graft Fenestrated One Endovascular (L)
O20.3	Placement Stent Graft One Endovascular NEC (L)
O20.5	Placement Stent Graft Three Endovascular (L)
O20.4	Placement Stent Graft Two Endovascular (L)
L76.-	Placement Stent Metallic Endovascular
L89.-	Placement Stent Other Endovascular
L76.-	Placement Stent Plastic Endovascular
A11.2	Placement Surface Electrodes Electroencephalography
N08.-	Placement Testis Scrotum Bilateral
N09.-	Placement Testis Scrotum NEC
Z45.4	Placenta site
X48.-	Plaster Cast
	Plastic Reconstruction – see Reconstruction site Plastic
	Plastic Repair – see Repair site Plastic
S23.-	Plasty W
S23.-	Plasty Z
W19.1	Plating & Pinning Femur Neck Fracture NEC
T10.-	Pleura Operations Endoscopic Therapeutic
T14.-	Pleura Operations NEC
T09.-	Pleura Operations Open NEC
Z52.1	Pleura site
T13.-	Pleural Cavity Introduction Substance
T14.-	Pleural Cavity Operations NEC
Z52.2	Pleural Cavity site
T07.-	Pleurectomy
T10.-	Pleurodesis Access Minimal
T10.-	Pleurodesis Endoscopic
T09.-	Pleurodesis Open
	Plication – see also Tucking
H42.2	Plication Anal Sphincter & Muscle Levator Ani Perineal
W81.6	Plication Capsule Joint

T16.2	Plication Diaphragm
C33.-	Plication Eye Muscle
G46.1	Plication Gastro-oesophageal Junction Endoluminal Endoscopic Fibreoptic
N11.2	Plication Hydrocele Sac
G76.4	Plication Ileum
M05.4	Plication Kidney
C33.-	Plication Muscle Eye
H42.2	Plication Muscle Levator Ani & Anal Sphincter Perineal
N28.3	Plication Penis Corpora
Q54.2	Plication Uterus Ligament Round
L79.2	Plication Vena Cava
E54.-	Pneumonectomy
F16.7	Polishing Teeth
W01.2	Pollicisation Finger
	Polypectomy – see also Excision Lesion
E08.1	Polypectomy Nose Internal
U33.1	Polysomnography
Z22.6	Postnasal Space site
P31.-	Pouch Douglas Operations
Z44.6	Pouch Douglas site
X68.-	Preparation Brachytherapy
X67.-	Preparation Radiotherapy External Beam
F17.6	Preparation Teeth Bridge
F17.1	Preparation Tooth Crown Dental
F11.-	Preprosthetic Oral Surgery
N30.-	Prepuce Operations
Z42.6	Prepuce site
N30.-	Prepuce Skin Operations
Z42.6	Prepuce Skin site
N30.1	Prepuceplasty
E85.2	Pressure Airway Continuous Positive Support
E85.2	Pressure Chest-wall Continuous Negative Support
	Pressure Monitoring – see Manometry
Y70.4	Primary Operations NOC
C27.5	Probing Nasolacrimal Duct NEC
H55.6	Probing Perineal Fistula
	Procedures – see Operation site
M33.-	Procedures Ureter Stent Percutaneous
H33.2	Proctectomy & Anastomosis Colon Anus
H41.4	Proctectomy Mucosal Peranal & Anastomosis Endoanal
H04.1	Proctocolectomy NEC
H62.6	Proctoscopy
X70.-	Procurement Chemotherapy Neoplasm Drugs Bands 1-5
X71.-	Procurement Chemotherapy Neoplasm Drugs Bands 6-10
L60.-	Profundoplasty Artery Femoral
L60.-	Profundoplasty Artery Popliteal
M67.-	Prostate Operations Endoscopic Therapeutic NEC
M62.-	Prostate Operations Open NEC
M71.-	Prostate Operations Other NEC
Z42.2	Prostate site

M67.5	Prostatectomy Microwave Endoscopic
M61.-	Prostatectomy NEC
M62.3	Prostatotomy
	Prosthesis – see also Replacement
Y03.6	Prosthesis Adjustment NOC
G25.2	Prosthesis Angelchick Adjustment
G24.6	Prosthesis Angelchick Insertion
G25.3	Prosthesis Angelchick Removal
L22.-	Prosthesis Aorta Attention
L74.1	Prosthesis Arteriovenous Insertion
K43.-	Prosthesis Artery Coronary
Y03.-	Prosthesis Attention NOC
J40.-	Prosthesis Bile Duct Endoscopic Retrograde
J47.-	Prosthesis Bile Duct Insertion Percutaneous
J48.-	Prosthesis Bile Duct Insertion Percutaneous Attention
J31.-	Prosthesis Bile Duct Open
M55.-	Prosthesis Bladder Outlet Female Collar
M64.-	Prosthesis Bladder Outlet Male Collar
O09.-	Prosthesis Bone (W)
H24.3	Prosthesis Bowel Lower Tubal Insertion Sigmoidoscope Fibreoptic
B30.-	Prosthesis Breast
B30.4	Prosthesis Breast Renewal
T02.-	Prosthesis Chest Wall
D24.-	Prosthesis Cochlear
H24.3	Prosthesis Colon Sigmoid Tubal Insertion Endoscopic NEC
H24.3	Prosthesis Colon Sigmoid Tubal Insertion Sigmoidoscope Fibreoptic
H27.3	Prosthesis Colon Sigmoid Tubal Insertion Sigmoidoscope Rigid
H24.3	Prosthesis Colon Tubal Insertion Sigmoidoscope Fibreoptic
C40.4	Prosthesis Conjunctiva
Y03.5	Prosthesis Conversion NOC
C46.4	Prosthesis Cornea Insertion
Y03.3	Prosthesis Correction Displaced NOC
V01.4	Prosthesis Cranium Removal
F63.-	Prosthesis Dental
T16.1	Prosthesis Diaphragm Repair
G44.1	Prosthesis Duodenum Proximal Insertion & Exam. U.G.I. Tract Endoscope Fibreoptic
G44.1	Prosthesis Duodenum Proximal Insertion & Exam. U.G.I. Tract Endoscope NEC
G54.3	Prosthesis Duodenum Tubal Insertion Endoscopic NEC
G53.4	Prosthesis Duodenum Tubal Insertion Open
C04.-	Prosthesis Eye Attention
C03.-	Prosthesis Eye Insertion
C23.2	Prosthesis Eyelid Upper Weight
Q26.-	Prosthesis Fallopian Tube
G44.1	Prosthesis Gastrointestinal Tract Upper Insertion Endoscope Fibreoptic
G44.1	Prosthesis Gastrointestinal Tract Upper Insertion Endoscopic NEC
K02.-	Prosthesis Heart
J40.-	Prosthesis Hepatic Duct Endoscopic Retrograde
J47.-	Prosthesis Hepatic Duct Insertion Percutaneous
J31.-	Prosthesis Hepatic Duct Open
J29.-	Prosthesis Hepatic Duct Open & Anastomosis Jejunum

G79.3	Prosthesis Ileum Tubal Insertion Endoscopic
G79.3	Prosthesis Intestine Small Tubal Insertion Endoscopic NEC
G64.3	Prosthesis Jejunum Tubal Insertion Endoscopic
	Prosthesis Joint – see Replacement Joint
M06.4	Prosthesis Kidney Attention
E31.-	Prosthesis Larynx
E31.3	Prosthesis Larynx Insertion & Division Stenosis
E35.4	Prosthesis Larynx Removal Endoscopic
C75.-	Prosthesis Lens
X05.-	Prosthesis Limb Attention
X05.-	Prosthesis Limb Implantation
J15.-	Prosthesis Liver Blood Vessel Insertion Transluminal
Y03.1	Prosthesis Maintenance NOC
Y02.-	Prosthesis NOC
E03.7	Prosthesis Nose Septum Perforation
G44.1	Prosthesis Oesophagus Insertion & Exam. U.G.I. Tract Endoscopic Fibreoptic
G44.1	Prosthesis Oesophagus Insertion & Exam. U.G.I. Tract Endoscopic NEC
G11.-	Prosthesis Oesophagus Open
G15.4	Prosthesis Oesophagus Tubal Insertion Endoscopic Fibreoptic
G18.4	Prosthesis Oesophagus Tubal Insertion Endoscopic NEC
C03.-	Prosthesis Orbit
C04.-	Prosthesis Orbit Attention
C04.-	Prosthesis Orbit Revision
D16.-	Prosthesis Ossicular Chain
J42.-	Prosthesis Pancreatic Duct Endoscopic Retrograde
J60.-	Prosthesis Pancreatic Duct Tubal Insertion
N29.-	Prosthesis Penis
M68.-	Prosthesis Prostate Insertion Endoscopic
G44.1	Prosthesis Pylorus Insertion Endoscopic Fibreoptic
G44.1	Prosthesis Pylorus Insertion Endoscopic NEC
H24.3	Prosthesis Rectum Tubal Insertion Endoscopic NEC
H24.3	Prosthesis Rectum Tubal Insertion Sigmoidoscope Fibreoptic
H27.3	Prosthesis Rectum Tubal Insertion Sigmoidoscope Rigid
Y03.7	Prosthesis Removal NOC
Y03.2	Prosthesis Renewal NOC
Y03.4	Prosthesis Resiting NOC
O09.1	Prosthesis Rib Vertical Expanding Titanium (W)
C54.-	Prosthesis Sclera for Attachment of Retina Attention
G44.1	Prosthesis Stomach Insertion Endoscopic Fibreoptic
G44.1	Prosthesis Stomach Insertion Endoscopic NEC
G38.2	Prosthesis Stomach Insertion Open
G18.4	Prosthesis Stomach Tubal Insertion Gastroscope Rigid
T74.2	Prosthesis Tendon Removal
N10.-	Prosthesis Testis
E41.-	Prosthesis Trachea
M29.-	Prosthesis Ureter Tubal Endoscopic NEC
M26.4	Prosthesis Ureter Tubal Insertion Nephroscopic
M29.5	Prosthesis Ureter Tubal Renewal Endoscopic
M75.2	Prosthesis Urethra Bulb Male Compression
L73.-	Protection Blood Vessel Mechanical Embolic

Z75.5	Pubis Ramus site
M73.5	Pull Through Urethra
	Pump – see also Cannulation
Y73.1	Pump Cardiovascular
	Puncture – see also Drainage
	Puncture – see also Injection
W36.-	Puncture Bone Diagnostic
W36.-	Puncture Bone NEC
W36.-	Puncture Bone Percutaneous NEC
W35.5	Puncture Bone Percutaneous Therapeutic
W35.-	Puncture Bone Therapeutic
A22.2	Puncture Brain Cistern
A10.5	Puncture Brain Tissue NEC
W90.-	Puncture Joint
M13.-	Puncture Kidney Pelvis Percutaneous
M13.-	Puncture Kidney Percutaneous
J14.-	Puncture Liver NEC
A55.9	Puncture Lumbar NEC
E13.6	Puncture Maxillary Antrum
Y33.-	Puncture NOC
J67.2	Puncture Pancreatic Duct Percutaneous & Pancreatography
T12.-	Puncture Pleura
A55.-	Puncture Spinal Diagnostic
A54.-	Puncture Spinal Therapeutic
W36.4	Puncture Sternum Diagnostic
E41.4	Puncture Tracheo-oesophageal Speech Prosthesis Insertion
A20.8	Puncture Ventricle NEC
C60.4	Pupilloplasty
M13.5	Pyelography Antegrade
X31.2	Pyelography Intravenous
M30.1	Pyelography Retrograde Endoscopic
M06.1	Pyelolithotomy
M10.2	Pyeloplasty Endoscopic
M05.-	Pyeloplasty Open
M12.1	Pyeloureterodynamics Percutaneous
G40.1	Pyloromyotomy
G40.-	Pyloroplasty
G41.-	Pylorus Operations NEC
Z27.3	Pylorus site

Q

B28.1	Quadrantectomy Breast
T79.2	Quadricepsplasty

R

	Radical Operations – refer to Tabular List Introduction
A55.1	Radiculography
A55.1	Radiculography Lumbar
Y35.-	Radioactive Material Removable Introduction NOC
Y36.3	Radioactive Seed Implantation NEC
Y53.1	Radiological Control Approach
U08.-	Radiology Abdomen Diagnostic
U04.1	Radiology Bitewing
U05.-	Radiology Central Nervous System Diagnostic
U07.-	Radiology Chest Diagnostic
Y97.-	Radiology Contrast
U06.-	Radiology Face & Neck Diagnostic
K63.-	Radiology Heart Contrast
U10.-	Radiology Heart Diagnostic
U04.4	Radiology Jaw Lateral Oblique
T90.-	Radiology Lymphatic Tissue Contrast
U13.-	Radiology Musculoskeletal Diagnostic
U04.3	Radiology Occlusal
U09.-	Radiology Pelvis Diagnostic
U04.2	Radiology Periapical
Y98.-	Radiology Procedures
U12.-	Radiology Urinary Diagnostic
U11.-	Radiology Vascular Diagnostic
A10.7	Radiosurgery Brain Tissue Stereotactic
C39.5	Radiotherapy Conjunctiva Lesion
C45.5	Radiotherapy Cornea Lesion
X65.-	Radiotherapy Delivery
Y91.-	Radiotherapy External Beam
C24.2	Radiotherapy Lacrimal Gland
J12.3	Radiotherapy Liver Lesion Selective Internal Using Microspheres
Y90.2	Radiotherapy NEC
A61.3	Radiotherapy Nerve Peripheral Lesion
C82.3	Radiotherapy Retina Lesion External Beam
C82.3	Radiotherapy Retina Lesion NEC
C82.4	Radiotherapy Retina Lesion Plaque
Z72.1	Radius & Ulna Shaft Combination site
Z70.-	Radius site NEC
	Re-excision – see also Excision
B28.4	Re-excision Breast Margins
T60.-	Re-excision Ganglion

S06.6	Re-excision Skin Margins Head Neck
S06.7	Re-excision Skin Margins NEC
	Re-exploration – see also Exploration
	Re-exploration – see also Reopening
Y32.-	Re-exploration & Arrest Bleeding Postoperative Surgical NOC
Y32.-	Re-exploration & Packing NOC
Y32.-	Re-exploration & Repair NOC
Y32.-	Re-exploration NOC
E94.3	Reactivity Bronchial
X12.-	Reamputation
J32.2	Reanastomosis Bile Duct
Q29.1	Reanastomosis Fallopian Tube NEC
H50.4	Reanastomosis Rectum Anal Canal Correction Rectum Atresia Congenital
	Reattachment – see also Repair
W84.-	Reattachment Ligament Intra-articular Endoscopic
W84.-	Reattachment Ligament Knee Intra-articular Endoscopic
Y04.1	Reattachment Microvascular NOC
H62.1	Recanalisation Bowel Laser NEC
Q41.6	Recanalisation Fallopian Tube
C31.-	Recession Eye Muscle & Resection
C31.-	Recession Eye Muscle Bilateral
C32.-	Recession Eye Muscle NEC
C17.3	Recession Eyelid Lower
C17.2	Recession Eyelid Upper
C31.-	Recession Muscle Eye & Resection
C31.-	Recession Muscle Eye Bilateral
C32.-	Recession Muscle Eye NEC
	Reconstruction – see also Refashioning
	Reconstruction – see also Reformation
L65.1	Reconstruction Aorta Revision
K17.3	Reconstruction Aortopulmonary Procedure
B36.-	Reconstruction Areola
L37.-	Reconstruction Artery Axillary
L37.8	Reconstruction Artery Axillary Graft
L37.-	Reconstruction Artery Brachial
L37.8	Reconstruction Artery Brachial Graft
L29.-	Reconstruction Artery Carotid
L34.1	Reconstruction Artery Cerebral
L34.1	Reconstruction Artery Circle Willis
L45.-	Reconstruction Artery Coeliac
L60.-	Reconstruction Artery Femoral
L65.3	Reconstruction Artery Femoral Revision
L52.-	Reconstruction Artery Iliac
L65.2	Reconstruction Artery Iliac Revision
L45.-	Reconstruction Artery Mesenteric
L60.-	Reconstruction Artery Popliteal
L65.3	Reconstruction Artery Popliteal Revision
L41.-	Reconstruction Artery Renal
L65.-	Reconstruction Artery Revision
L66.2	Reconstruction Artery Stent Transluminal Percutaneous

L37.-	Reconstruction Artery Subclavian
L37.8	Reconstruction Artery Subclavian Graft
L45.-	Reconstruction Artery Suprarenal
L37.-	Reconstruction Artery Vertebral
L37.8	Reconstruction Artery Vertebral Graft
K05.-	Reconstruction Atrium Transposition Arteries Great
D08.2	Reconstruction Auditory Canal External
J32.1	Reconstruction Bile Duct
M37.8	Reconstruction Bladder NEC
M54.2	Reconstruction Bladder Neck Female NEC
M64.6	Reconstruction Bladder Neck Male NEC
V13.1	Reconstruction Bone Face
W17.-	Reconstruction Bone NEC
W17.5	Reconstruction Bone Revision
B29.-	Reconstruction Breast
B39.-	Reconstruction Breast Flap Abdominal
B39.5	Reconstruction Breast Flap Free Omental
B39.4	Reconstruction Breast Flap Pedicled Omental
B39.3	Reconstruction Breast Free Flap Deep Inferior Epigastric Perforator
B39.1	Reconstruction Breast Free Flap Transverse Rectus Abdominis Myocutaneous
B39.2	Reconstruction Breast Pedicled Flap Transverse Rectus Abdominis Myocutaneous
B29.5	Reconstruction Breast Revision
B38.-	Reconstruction Breast Skin Flap Buttock
E44.-	Reconstruction Carina
W02.-	Reconstruction Carpus
T02.-	Reconstruction Chest Wall
X21.7	Reconstruction Club Hand Radial
V02.3	Reconstruction Cranium NEC
D03.-	Reconstruction Ear External
D03.-	Reconstruction Ear External Skin
C14.-	Reconstruction Eyelid
Q30.1	Reconstruction Fallopian Tube
W03.-	Reconstruction Forefoot Complex
W02.-	Reconstruction Hand Complex NEC
W02.-	Reconstruction Hand Soft Tissue Complex NEC
W04.-	Reconstruction Hindfoot Complex
V19.1	Reconstruction Jaw NEC
W57.-	Reconstruction Joint Excision
W02.-	Reconstruction Joint Hand Multiple NEC
W56.-	Reconstruction Joint Interposition Natural Tissue
W56.-	Reconstruction Joint Interposition NEC
W55.-	Reconstruction Joint Interposition Prosthetic
W58.-	Reconstruction Joint NEC
O10.-	Reconstruction Joint Shoulder Complex (W)
V20.-	Reconstruction Joint Temporomandibular
E31.1	Reconstruction Laryngotracheal Graft Cartilage
E31.-	Reconstruction Larynx
W77.6	Reconstruction Ligament Annular
O27.1	Reconstruction Ligament Extra-articular Stabilisation Joint (W)
W74.-	Reconstruction Ligament NEC

F04.-	Reconstruction Lip NEC
F04.-	Reconstruction Lip Skin NEC
T89.1	Reconstruction Lymphatic Duct
V19.1	Reconstruction Mandible
Y24.1	Reconstruction Microvascular NOC
F39.-	Reconstruction Mouth NEC
B36.-	Reconstruction Nipple
Y26.1	Reconstruction NOC
E02.-	Reconstruction Nose
C05.1	Reconstruction Orbit Cavity
D16.-	Reconstruction Ossicular Chain
N28.2	Reconstruction Penis
N03.6	Reconstruction Scrotum
V12.5	Reconstruction Skull NEC
T72.1	Reconstruction Tendon Sheath
W01.-	Reconstruction Thumb
W01.-	Reconstruction Thumb Complex
E40.-	Reconstruction Trachea
M73.4	Reconstruction Urethra
P32.1	Reconstruction Vagina Interposition Bowel
P21.2	Reconstruction Vagina NEC
P32.2	Reconstruction Vagina Pelvic Peritoneal Graft
P32.3	Reconstruction Vagina Urethral Dissection
L99.2	Reconstruction Vein Stent Transluminal Percutaneous
U19.5	Recording Holter Extended Electrocardiographic
F42.5	Recording Jaw Relationships
Z29.4	Rectosigmoid site
H33.-	Rectosigmoidectomy
H33.3	Rectosigmoidectomy & Anastomosis Colon
H41.1	Rectosigmoidectomy & Anastomosis Peranal
H33.5	Rectosigmoidectomy & Closure Rectal Stump & Exteriorisation Bowel
H42.-	Rectum Mucosa Prolapse Operations Perineal
H27.-	Rectum Operations Endoscopic NEC
H27.-	Rectum Operations Endoscopic Sigmoidoscope Rigid NEC
	Rectum Operations NEC – see also Bowel Operations NEC
H46.-	Rectum Operations NEC
H24.-	Rectum Operations Therapeutic Sigmoidoscope Fibreoptic NEC
H40.-	Rectum Operations Through Anal Sphincter
H41.-	Rectum Operations Through Anus NEC
H36.-	Rectum Prolapse Operations Abdominal NEC
H42.-	Rectum Prolapse Operations Perineal
Z29.1	Rectum site
D05.3	Reduction Auricular Soft Tissue Prosthesis
V09.-	Reduction Bone Face Fracture NEC
W25.-	Reduction Bone Fracture Closed & Fixation External
W24.-	Reduction Bone Fracture Closed & Fixation Internal
W24.6	Reduction Bone Fracture Closed & Fixation Nail or Screw
W26.-	Reduction Bone Fracture Closed NEC
O17.-	Reduction Bone Fracture Closed Secondary & Fixation Internal (W)
W21.-	Reduction Bone Fracture Intra-articular Open

W19.-	Reduction Bone Fracture Open & Fixation Intramedullary
W20.-	Reduction Bone Fracture Open & Fixation NEC
W22.-	Reduction Bone Fracture Open NEC
W19.-	Reduction Bone Fracture Open Primary & Fixation Intramedullary
W20.-	Reduction Bone Fracture Open Primary & Fixation NEC
W22.-	Reduction Bone Fracture Open Primary NEC
W23.-	Reduction Bone Fracture Open Secondary
W24.-	Reduction Bone Fragment Closed & Fixation
O17.5	Reduction Bone Fragment Closed Secondary & Fixation Internal (W)
W19.-	Reduction Bone Fragment Open & Fixation
D13.3	Reduction Bone Mastoid Soft Tissue Prosthesis Anchored Hearing
V09.-	Reduction Bone Nose Fracture
H17.1	Reduction Caecum Intussusception Open
H17.2	Reduction Caecum Volvulus Open
P01.2	Reduction Clitoris
H17.1	Reduction Colon Intussusception Open
H30.1	Reduction Colon Intussusception Radiological Enema Barium
H30.3	Reduction Colon Sigmoid Volvulus Flatus Tube
H17.3	Reduction Colon Sigmoid Volvulus Open
H17.4	Reduction Colon Volvulus Open NEC
	Reduction Dislocation – see Reduction Joint
W48.5	Reduction Femur Head Prosthesis Dislocated Closed
X25.3	Reduction Foot Gigantism
	Reduction Fracture – see Reduction Bone
G44.4	Reduction Gastroenterostomy Intussusception Endoscopic Fibreoptic
G33.4	Reduction Gastroenterostomy Intussusception Open
	Reduction Gigantism – see Reduction site
H53.3	Reduction Haemorrhoid Prolapsed Manual
X21.1	Reduction Hand Gigantism
G75.5	Reduction Ileostomy Prolapse
G76.1	Reduction Ileum Intussusception Open
G82.1	Reduction Ileum Intussusception Radiological Enema Barium
G82.1	Reduction Intestine Small Intussusception Radiol. Enema Barium NEC
V15.-	Reduction Jaw Fracture NEC
W66.-	Reduction Joint Dislocation Closed
W66.4	Reduction Joint Dislocation Fracture Closed Primary & Fixation Internal
W66.-	Reduction Joint Dislocation Manipulative
W66.-	Reduction Joint Dislocation NEC
W65.-	Reduction Joint Dislocation Open
W67.-	Reduction Joint Dislocation Secondary
	Reduction Joint Fracture Dislocation – see Reduction Joint Dislocation
W68.-	Reduction Joint Growth Plate Injury
X22.1	Reduction Joint Hip Deformity Congenital Open
W39.6	Reduction Joint Hip Prosthesis Dislocated Closed
X23.1	Reduction Joint Knee Dislocation Congenital Operative
V21.2	Reduction Joint Temporomandibular Dislocation
P05.7	Reduction Labia Major
P05.6	Reduction Labia Minor
V15.-	Reduction Mandible Fracture
V08.-	Reduction Maxilla Fracture

E04.2	Reduction Nose Turbinate NEC
C08.-	Reduction Orbit Fracture
N30.6	Reduction Prepuce Manual
H46.-	Reduction Rectum Intussusception
H44.2	Reduction Rectum Prolapse Manual
A49.4	Reduction Spinal Cord Abnormal Tissue Complex
V45.-	Reduction Spine Fracture NEC
X19.1	Reduction Sprengel Deformity
G38.6	Reduction Stomach Volvulus
N13.3	Reduction Testis Torsion
	Refashioning – see also Operation site
	Refashioning – see also Revision
K20.-	Refashioning Atrium
S60.4	Refashioning Scar NEC
Y03.1	Refilling Pump NOC
C69.1	Reformation Eye Anterior Chamber
U52.2	Rehabilitation Addiction Alcohol
U52.1	Rehabilitation Addiction Drug
U51.1	Rehabilitation Brain Injuries
U53.3	Rehabilitation Burns
U54.1	Rehabilitation Cardiac Disorders
U50.2	Rehabilitation Hip Fracture
U50.3	Rehabilitation Joint Replacement
U50.1	Rehabilitation Limb Amputation
U50.-	Rehabilitation Musculoskeletal Disorders
U54.1	Rehabilitation Myocardial Infarction Acute
U51.-	Rehabilitation Neurological Disorders
U50.5	Rehabilitation Osteoarthritis
U54.-	Rehabilitation Other Disorders
U51.3	Rehabilitation Pain Syndromes
U52.-	Rehabilitation Psychiatric Disorders
U53.-	Rehabilitation Reconstructive Surgery
U54.2	Rehabilitation Respiratory Disorders
U50.4	Rehabilitation Rheumatoid Arthritis
U51.2	Rehabilitation Spinal Cord Injury
U54.3	Rehabilitation Stroke
U53.-	Rehabilitation Trauma
	Reimplantation – see Replantation
W73.-	Reinforcement Ligament Prosthetic
S23.-	Relaxation Skin Contracture Operations Flap
X61.2	Relaxation Therapy Session
	Release Adhesions – see Freeing site Adhesions
L23.4	Release Aorta Vascular Ring
V02.1	Release Calvarium Posterior
A65.2	Release Canal Guyon
A65.1	Release Carpal Tunnel
A69.2	Release Carpal Tunnel Revision
A67.1	Release Cubital Tunnel
T51.-	Release Fascia Abdomen
T55.-	Release Fascia NEC

T51.2	Release Fascia Pelvis
X24.-	Release Foot Joint Correction Foot Deformity Congenital
W04.5	Release Hindfoot Soft Tissue
W78.4	Release Joint Capsule Contracture Limited
W78.-	Release Joint Contracture
T80.-	Release Muscle Contracture
T80.4	Release Muscle Sternomastoid
T80.-	Release Muscle Tether
T80.3	Release Neck Webbing
A31.-	Release Nerve Cranial Intracranial Stereotactic
A67.2	Release Nerve Lateral Cutaneous Thigh Entrapment
A66.-	Release Nerve Peripheral Ankle Entrapment
A67.-	Release Nerve Peripheral Entrapment NEC
A68.-	Release Nerve Peripheral NEC
A69.-	Release Nerve Peripheral Revision
A65.-	Release Nerve Peripheral Wrist Entrapment
A67.3	Release Nerve Plantar Digital Entrapment
Y18.-	Release NOC
X20.-	Release Radius Correction Forearm Deformity Congenital
V42.3	Release Spine Anterolateral & Graft
X27.1	Release Streeter Band
A66.1	Release Tarsal Tunnel
A69.3	Release Tarsal Tunnel Revision
T72.3	Release Tendon Sheath Constriction
T80.2	Release Tether Cicatricial
T80.1	Release Tether Paralytic
X27.2	Release Toe Syndactyly
F26.3	Release Tongue Tie
T80.4	Release Torticollis
X20.-	Release Ulna Correction Forearm Deformity Congenital
H17.6	Relief Caecum Obstruction Open NEC
H17.5	Relief Caecum Strangulation Open
H17.6	Relief Colon Obstruction Open NEC
H17.5	Relief Colon Strangulation Open
G76.3	Relief Ileum Obstruction Open NEC
G76.2	Relief Ileum Strangulation Open
K24.-	Relief Ventricular Outflow Tract Obstruction
W25.-	Remanipulation Bone Fracture
O17.-	Remanipulation Bone Fracture Closed & Fixation Internal (W)
W67.-	Remanipulation Joint Dislocation Fracture
W67.-	Remanipulation Joint Dislocation NEC
V02.2	Remodelling & Expansion Calvarium
V02.2	Remodelling Calvarium
V12.2	Remodelling Cranium & Bones Face
V12.1	Remodelling Cranium & Orbits
V12.1	Remodelling Fronto-orbital
	Removal – see also Excision
	Removal – see also Primary Operation site
	Removal – see also Removal from site
H57.3	Removal Anal Sphincter Artificial NEC

S63.3	Removal Autologous Bone Flap from Subcutaneous Storage Pocket
S63.3	Removal Autologous Tissue from Subcutaneous Storage Pocket
M60.2	Removal Balloon Male Continence Adjustable
U33.3	Removal Blood Pressure Monitor Ambulatory
	Removal Bypass – see Bypass site
K55.3	Removal Cardiac Thrombus Open
K55.4	Removal Cardiac Vegetations Open NEC
K59.5	Removal Cardioverter Defibrillator
K72.4	Removal Cardioverter Defibrillator Subcutaneous
Q12.3	Removal Contraceptive Device Displaced NEC
P31.5	Removal Contraceptive Device Displaced Pouch Douglas
Q12.4	Removal Contraceptive Device Uterine Cavity
U19.7	Removal Electrocardiography Loop Recorder
	Removal Explant – see Explant site
	Removal Fixation – see Fixation site
	Removal Foreign Body – see also Removal from site Foreign Body
Y29.-	Removal Foreign Body NOC
	Removal from – see also Evacuation
T31.6	Removal from Abdominal Wall Anterior Foreign Body
T31.6	Removal from Abdominal Wall Foreign Body NEC
T39.8	Removal from Abdominal Wall Posterior Foreign Body
D07.3	Removal from Auditory Canal External Foreign Body
D07.2	Removal from Auditory Canal External Wax NEC
J41.1	Removal from Bile Duct Calculus Endoscopic Retrograde
J33.-	Removal from Bile Duct Calculus Open
J49.-	Removal from Bile Duct Calculus T Tube Track Endoscopic
J49.-	Removal from Bile Duct Calculus T Tube Track Percutaneous
J76.1	Removal from Bile Duct Calculus Transhepatic Percutaneous
M44.4	Removal from Bladder Blood Clot Endoscopic
M44.2	Removal from Bladder Calculus Endoscopic NEC
M39.1	Removal from Bladder Calculus Open
M44.3	Removal from Bladder Foreign Body Endoscopic
M39.2	Removal from Bladder Foreign Body Open
M55.7	Removal from Bladder Outlet Female Balloon Continence Adjustable
M55.7	Removal from Bladder Outlet Female Device Retropubic
M54.3	Removal from Bladder Outlet Female Urinary Sphincter Artificial
M60.3	Removal from Bladder Outlet Male Urinary Sphincter Artificial
M49.3	Removal from Bladder Suprapubic Tube
W35.3	Removal from Bone Substance Implanted
A07.2	Removal from Brain Tissue Foreign Body
E48.5	Removal from Bronchus Foreign Body Endoscopic NEC
E50.5	Removal from Bronchus Foreign Body Endoscopic Rigid
H21.3	Removal from Caecum Foreign Body Endoscopic Fibreoptic
H21.3	Removal from Caecum Foreign Body Endoscopic NEC
H19.4	Removal from Caecum Foreign Body Open
E48.5	Removal from Carina Foreign Body Endoscopic NEC
E50.5	Removal from Carina Foreign Body Endoscopic Rigid
T01.2	Removal from Chest Wall Plombage
T05.4	Removal from Chest Wall Wire
H21.3	Removal from Colon Foreign Body Endoscopic Fibreoptic

H21.3	Removal from Colon Foreign Body Endoscopic NEC
H19.4	Removal from Colon Foreign Body Open
H24.8	Removal from Colon Sigmoid Foreign Body Endoscopic NEC
H27.2	Removal from Colon Sigmoid Foreign Body Sigmoidoscope Rigid
H31.5	Removal from Colorectum Stent Image Guided
C43.3	Removal from Conjunctiva Foreign Body
C48.-	Removal from Cornea Foreign Body
G54.8	Removal from Duodenum Foreign Body Endoscopic NEC
G53.3	Removal from Duodenum Foreign Body Open
G44.2	Removal from Duodenum Prox. Foreign Body & Exam. U.G.I. Tract Endo. NEC
G44.2	Removal from Duodenum Prox. Foreign Body & Exam. U.G.I. Tract Fibreoptic
D05.7	Removal from Ear External Hearing Implant
D20.6	Removal from Ear Middle Hearing Implant
C86.4	Removal from Eye Foreign Body NEC
C22.3	Removal from Eyelid Foreign Body
C23.3	Removal from Eyelid Upper Weight
Q37.1	Removal from Fallopian Tube Clip Access Minimal
Q37.1	Removal from Fallopian Tube Clip Endoscopic
Q29.2	Removal from Fallopian Tube Clip Open NEC
Q31.1	Removal from Fallopian Tube Products Conception NEC
Q29.2	Removal from Fallopian Tube Ring Open NEC
J08.1	Removal from Gall Bladder Calculus Access Minimal
J08.1	Removal from Gall Bladder Calculus Endoscopic NEC
J08.1	Removal from Gall Bladder Calculus Laparoscopic
J21.1	Removal from Gall Bladder Calculus Open
J08.1	Removal from Gall Bladder Calculus Peritoneoscope
G44.2	Removal from Gastrointestinal Tract Upper Foreign Body Endoscopic Fibreoptic
G44.2	Removal from Gastrointestinal Tract Upper Foreign Body Endoscopic NEC
K57.3	Removal from Heart Foreign Body Transluminal Percutaneous
K55.3	Removal from Heart Thrombus
K37.-	Removal from Heart Valve Structure Adjacent Obstruction
K55.4	Removal from Heart Vegetations
T27.-	Removal from Hernia Abdominal Wall Material Prosthetic Repair NEC
T23.4	Removal from Hernia Femoral Material Prosthetic Repair
T26.4	Removal from Hernia Incisional Material Prosthetic Repair
T21.4	Removal from Hernia Inguinal Material Prosthetic Repair
T24.4	Removal from Hernia Umbilical Material Prosthetic Repair
T27.4	Removal from Hernia Ventral Material Prosthetic Repair
G78.3	Removal from Ileum Foreign Body
G78.3	Removal from Intestine Small Foreign Body NEC
C64.5	Removal from Iris Foreign Body
W85.1	Removal from Joint Knee Loose Body Endoscopic
W86.1	Removal from Joint Loose Body Endoscopic NEC
W81.2	Removal from Joint Loose Body Open
M09.4	Removal from Kidney Calculus Endoscopic NEC
M06.1	Removal from Kidney Calculus Open
M06.1	Removal from Kidney Pelvis Calculus Open
E35.5	Removal from Larynx Foreign Body Endoscopic
C77.-	Removal from Lens Foreign Body
J08.1	Removal from Liver Calculus Access Minimal

J08.1	Removal from Liver Calculus Endoscopic NEC
J08.1	Removal from Liver Calculus Laparoscope
J05.2	Removal from Liver Calculus Open
J12.2	Removal from Liver Calculus Percutaneous
J08.1	Removal from Liver Calculus Peritoneoscope
J04.1	Removal from Liver Fragment Lacerated
E48.5	Removal from Lung Foreign Body Endoscopic NEC
E50.5	Removal from Lung Foreign Body Endoscopic Rigid
F40.5	Removal from Mouth Suture NEC
S70.3	Removal from Nail Foreign Body
E27.4	Removal from Nasopharynx Foreign Body
E08.5	Removal from Nose Cavity Foreign Body
G44.2	Removal from Oesophagus Foreign Body & Exam. U.G.I. Tract Endoscopic NEC
G44.2	Removal from Oesophagus Foreign Body & Exam. U.G.I. Tract Fibreoptic Endoscopic
G15.1	Removal from Oesophagus Foreign Body Endoscopic Fibreoptic
G15.1	Removal from Oesophagus Foreign Body Endoscopic NEC
G15.1	Removal from Oesophagus Foreign Body NEC
G18.1	Removal from Oesophagus Foreign Body Oesophagoscope Rigid
G13.2	Removal from Oesophagus Foreign Body Open
C06.4	Removal from Orbit Foreign Body
Y44.4	Removal from Organ Calculus
F32.2	Removal from Palate Foreign Body
J60.-	Removal from Pancreatic Duct Calculus
J42.3	Removal from Pancreatic Duct Calculus Endoscopic Retrograde
F56.1	Removal from Parotid Duct Calculus Manipulative
F51.1	Removal from Parotid Duct Calculus Open
N32.5	Removal from Penis Constricting Object
T42.4	Removal from Peritoneum Foreign Body Access Minimal
T42.4	Removal from Peritoneum Foreign Body Endoscopic
T41.4	Removal from Peritoneum Foreign Body NEC
F36.4	Removal from Peritonsillar Region Foreign Body
E27.4	Removal from Pharynx Foreign Body
P31.5	Removal from Pouch Douglas Contraceptive Device Intrauterine
P31.6	Removal from Pouch Douglas Foreign Body NEC
M67.4	Removal from Prostate Calculus Endoscopic
M68.2	Removal from Prostate Stent Cystoscopic
G44.2	Removal from Pylorus Foreign Body Endoscopic Fibreoptic
G44.2	Removal from Pylorus Foreign Body Endoscopic NEC
H44.1	Removal from Rectum Foreign Body Manual
H27.2	Removal from Rectum Foreign Body Sigmoidoscope Rigid
E48.5	Removal from Respiratory Tract Lower Foreign Body Endoscopic NEC
E50.5	Removal from Respiratory Tract Lower Foreign Body Endoscopic Rigid
F56.-	Removal from Salivary Duct Calculus Manipulative
F51.-	Removal from Salivary Duct Calculus Open
N03.5	Removal from Scrotum Foreign Body
S54.2	Removal from Skin Burnt Slough Head
S55.2	Removal from Skin Burnt Slough NEC
S54.2	Removal from Skin Burnt Slough Neck
S43.-	Removal from Skin Clip
S44.-	Removal from Skin Foreign Body Inorganic NEC

S45.-	Removal from Skin Foreign Body NEC
S43.-	Removal from Skin Repair Material
S56.2	Removal from Skin Slough Head NEC
S57.2	Removal from Skin Slough NEC
S56.2	Removal from Skin Slough Neck NEC
S44.-	Removal from Skin Substance Inorganic NEC
S45.-	Removal from Skin Substance NEC
S43.-	Removal from Skin Suture
V18.5	Removal from Skull Distractor External
V18.6	Removal from Skull Distractor Internal
V18.6	Removal from Skull Spring
A45.5	Removal from Spinal Cord Foreign Body
A45.5	Removal from Spinal Tract Foreign Body
V46.5	Removal from Spine Fixation Device
V40.5	Removal from Spine Instrumentation
G44.2	Removal from Stomach Foreign Body Endoscopic Fibreoptic
G44.2	Removal from Stomach Foreign Body Endoscopic NEC
G18.1	Removal from Stomach Foreign Body Gastroscope Rigid
G38.4	Removal from Stomach Foreign Body Open
G38.7	Removal from Stomach Gastric Band
S54.2	Removal from Subcutaneous Tissue Burnt Slough Head
S55.2	Removal from Subcutaneous Tissue Burnt Slough NEC
S54.2	Removal from Subcutaneous Tissue Burnt Slough Neck
S43.-	Removal from Subcutaneous Tissue Clip
S63.1	Removal from Subcutaneous Tissue Device Diagnostic
S44.-	Removal from Subcutaneous Tissue Foreign Body Inorganic NEC
S45.-	Removal from Subcutaneous Tissue Foreign Body NEC
S62.5	Removal from Subcutaneous Tissue Implant Hormone
S62.4	Removal from Subcutaneous Tissue Pack
S43.-	Removal from Subcutaneous Tissue Repair Material
S56.2	Removal from Subcutaneous Tissue Slough Head NEC
S57.2	Removal from Subcutaneous Tissue Slough NEC
S56.2	Removal from Subcutaneous Tissue Slough Neck NEC
S44.-	Removal from Subcutaneous Tissue Substance Inorganic NEC
S62.3	Removal from Subcutaneous Tissue Substance Inserted NEC
S45.-	Removal from Subcutaneous Tissue Substance NEC
F56.2	Removal from Submandibular Duct Calculus Manipulative
N13.6	Removal from Testis Foreign Body
F24.2	Removal from Tongue Foreign Body
F36.4	Removal from Tonsil Foreign Body
E48.5	Removal from Trachea Foreign Body Endoscopic NEC
E50.5	Removal from Trachea Foreign Body Endoscopic Rigid
M28.-	Removal from Ureter Calculus Endoscopic NEC
M26.3	Removal from Ureter Calculus Nephroscopic
M27.3	Removal from Ureter Calculus Ureteroscopic
M22.2	Removal from Ureter Ligature
M33.6	Removal from Ureter Stent Percutaneous NEC
M27.5	Removal from Ureter Stent Ureteroscopic
M75.4	Removal from Urethra Calculus Open
M76.2	Removal from Urethra Foreign Body Endoscopic

M76.7	Removal from Urethra Stent Endoscopic
M86.1	Removal from Urinary Diversion Calculus Endoscopic
M83.3	Removal from Urinary Tract Foreign Body NEC
Q12.4	Removal from Uterine Cavity Contraceptive Device
Q15.4	Removal from Uterine Cavity Substance Therapeutic
R28.-	Removal from Uterus Delivered Products Conception Instrument
R29.-	Removal from Uterus Delivered Products Conception Manual
Q09.1	Removal from Uterus Products Conception Open
P29.4	Removal from Vagina Foreign Body
M53.5	Removal from Vagina Tension Free Tape Partial
M53.4	Removal from Vagina Tension Free Tape Total
L90.-	Removal from Vein Thrombus Open
L96.-	Removal from Vein Thrombus Percutaneous
L79.5	Removal from Vena Cava Filter
C79.7	Removal from Vitreous Body Internal Tamponade Agent
	Removal from Wound – see Removal from Skin
G38.7	Removal Gastric Band
	Removal Grommet – see Grommet site
	Removal Implant – see Implantation site
A54.5	Removal Intrathecal Drug Delivery Device Adjacent Spinal Cord
	Removal Ligature – see Ligature site
Y44.8	Removal Material Radioactive Removable NOC
E11.5	Removal Nasal Prosthesis Fixtures Attachment
F14.7	Removal Orthodontic Anchorage
F14.4	Removal Orthodontic Appliance NEC
F14.7	Removal Orthodontic Screw
	Removal Pack – see Packing
R29.1	Removal Placenta Uterus Delivered Manual
X48.3	Removal Plaster Cast
	Removal Prosthesis – see Prosthesis site
C80.6	Removal Retina Band
C80.6	Removal Retina Membrane NEC
C80.5	Removal Retina Membrane Vascular
M55.7	Removal Retropubic Device Female
M60.2	Removal Retropubic Male Device Continence
	Removal Shunt – see Shunt site
	Removal site – see Excision site
	Removal Snare – see Resection site
	Removal Spacer Prosthesis Joint – see Attention site Joint
H57.7	Removal Sphincter Dynamic Graciloplasty
A48.6	Removal Spinal Cord Adjacent Neurostimulator
	Removal Stent – see also Prosthesis
Y15.7	Removal Stent NOC
C80.6	Removal Subretinal Band
C80.6	Removal Subretinal Membrane NEC
C80.5	Removal Subretinal Vascular Membrane
	Removal Suture – see also Suture site
C65.4	Removal Suture Releasable Following Glaucoma Surgery
	Removal System – see System site
	Removal Tattoo – see Excision Skin Lesion

F17.5	Removal Tooth Crown Dental
F09.-	Removal Tooth Surgical
F09.-	Removal Tooth Wisdom
M53.7	Removal Transobturator Tape
	Removal Tube – see Drainage site
	Removal Tube – see Tube site
K54.2	Removal Ventricular Assist Device Open
	Removal Wire – see Removal from site
X40.-	Renal Failure Compensation NEC
Z41.4	Renal Pelvis site NEC
K72.3	Renewal Cardioverter Defibrillator Subcutaneous
	Renewal Pack – see Packing
	Renewal Prosthesis – see Prosthesis site
	Renewal Shunt – see Shunt site
	Renewal Stent – see Stent
Y15.2	Renewal Stent NOC
	Renewal Tube – see Tube
T05.8	Renewal Wire Chest Wall
U12.6	Renogram Mercaptoacetyltriglycine
U12.5	Renogram Static
	Reopening – see also Re-exploration
T30.-	Reopening Abdomen & Arrest Bleeding Intra-abdominal Postoperative Surgery
T30.-	Reopening Abdomen & Re-exploration Intra-abdominal Operation
T30.3	Reopening Abdomen NEC
T03.-	Reopening Chest & Arrest Bleeding Intrathoracic Postoperative Surgical
T03.-	Reopening Chest & Re-exploration Intrathoracic Operation
T03.-	Reopening Chest NEC
V03.-	Reopening Cranium
V03.-	Reopening Cranium & Arrest Bleeding Intracranial Postoperative Surg.
V03.-	Reopening Cranium & Re-exploration Intracranial Operation
E08.7	Reopening Nares Anterior Surgical
T30.3	Reopening Peritoneum NEC
	Repair – see also Closure
	Repair – see also Correction
T28.-	Repair Abdominal Wall NEC
T28.8	Repair Abdominal Wall with Prosthetic Insertion
H55.7	Repair Anal Fistula Plug
H50.-	Repair Anus
L23.-	Repair Aorta Plastic
L23.7	Repair Aortic Arch Interrupted
L23.-	Repair Aortic Coarctation
L23.-	Repair Aortic Hypoplasia
F15.6	Repair Appliance Orthodontic
L75.2	Repair Arteriovenous Fistula Acquired
L38.1	Repair Artery Axillary NEC
L38.1	Repair Artery Brachial NEC
L31.3	Repair Artery Carotid Endovascular
L30.1	Repair Artery Carotid NEC
K47.-	Repair Artery Coronary
K47.3	Repair Artery Coronary Aneurysmal

K47.2	Repair Artery Coronary Fistula Arteriovenous
K47.5	Repair Artery Coronary Malformation Arteriovenous
K47.4	Repair Artery Coronary Rupture
L62.1	Repair Artery Femoral NEC
K06.-	Repair Artery Great Transposition
L53.1	Repair Artery Iliac NEC
L68.-	Repair Artery NEC
L62.1	Repair Artery Popliteal NEC
L10.-	Repair Artery Pulmonary
L01.3	Repair Artery Pulmonary Origin Anomalous from Ascending Aorta
L10.4	Repair Artery Pulmonary Sling
L41.-	Repair Artery Renal
L38.1	Repair Artery Subclavian NEC
L38.1	Repair Artery Vertebral NEC
K22.2	Repair Atrium NEC
J32.-	Repair Bile Duct
K17.5	Repair Biventricular Hypoplastic Left Heart Syndrome
M37.-	Repair Bladder NEC
E47.3	Repair Bronchus NEC
C29.1	Repair Canaliculus
W82.3	Repair Cartilage Semilunar Endoscopic
W70.3	Repair Cartilage Semilunar NEC
Q05.1	Repair Cervix Uteri NEC
T05.3	Repair Chest Wall NEC
C40.-	Repair Conjunctiva
K20.3	Repair Cor Triatriatum
V12.4	Repair Craniofacial Cleft Subcranial
V12.3	Repair Craniofacial Cleft Transcranial
V05.4	Repair Cranium Fracture NEC
V02.3	Repair Cranium NEC
V01.-	Repair Cranium Plastic
V02.-	Repair Cranium Plastic Other
F63.4	Repair Denture
T16.-	Repair Diaphragm NEC
T15.-	Repair Diaphragm Rupture
G23.-	Repair Diaphragmatic Hernia
A39.-	Repair Dura
D06.-	Repair Ear External
D14.-	Repair Eardrum
P23.4	Repair Enterocele NEC
M73.2	Repair Epispadias
T28.1	Repair Exomphalos HFQ
C86.2	Repair Eye Injury Penetrating
C37.4	Repair Eye Muscle NEC
C17.-	Repair Eyelid NEC
C16.-	Repair Eyelid Plastic NEC
C17.-	Repair Eyelid Skin NEC
Q30.-	Repair Fallopian Tube NEC
T57.3	Repair Fascia
M37.5	Repair Fistula Bladder

M62.4	Repair Fistula Rectoprostatic
A06.4	Repair Fracture Cranium Growing
J20.-	Repair Gall Bladder
J20.3	Repair Gall Bladder Perforation
T28.1	Repair Gastroschisis HFQ
C86.2	Repair Globe
K55.6	Repair Heart Injury Traumatic
K17.-	Repair Heart Univentricular
K29.-	Repair Heart Valve Plastic NEC
K30.-	Repair Heart Valve Plastic Revision
K23.3	Repair Heart Wall NEC
L01.3	Repair Hemitruncus Arteriosus
T27.-	Repair Hernia Abdominal Wall NEC
T98.-	Repair Hernia Abdominal Wall Recurrent
T16.4	Repair Hernia Diaphragmatic Congenital
G23.-	Repair Hernia Diaphragmatic NEC
T22.-	Repair Hernia Femoral NEC
T23.-	Repair Hernia Femoral Recurrent
T25.-	Repair Hernia Incisional NEC
T26.-	Repair Hernia Incisional Recurrent
T20.-	Repair Hernia Inguinal NEC
T21.-	Repair Hernia Inguinal Recurrent
T25.-	Repair Hernia Parastomal NEC
T26.-	Repair Hernia Parastomal Recurrent
T24.-	Repair Hernia Umbilical
T97.-	Repair Hernia Umbilical Recurrent
T27.-	Repair Hernia Ventral
T98.1	Repair Hernia Ventral Insert Material Natural Recurrent
T98.2	Repair Hernia Ventral Insert Material Prosthetic Recurrent
T98.3	Repair Hernia Ventral Sutures Recurrent
P15.3	Repair Hymen
K17.-	Repair Hypoplastic Left Heart Syndrome
M73.1	Repair Hypospadias
G75.2	Repair Ileostomy Prolapse
P15.8	Repair Introitus
O27.-	Repair Joint Capsule Glenohumeral & Labrum (W)
W77.-	Repair Joint Capsule NEC
M05.-	Repair Kidney Open
W84.7	Repair Labrum Superior Tear Anterior Posterior Endoscopic
W84.-	Repair Ligament Intra-articular Endoscopic
W84.-	Repair Ligament Knee Intra-articular Endoscopic
W75.-	Repair Ligament NEC
W75.-	Repair Ligament Open
F05.-	Repair Lip NEC
F05.-	Repair Lip Skin NEC
J04.-	Repair Liver
E57.1	Repair Lung
A39.1	Repair Meningoencephalocele
A06.4	Repair Meningoencephalocele Post-traumatic
T38.4	Repair Mesentery Colon

T37.4	Repair Mesentery Intestine Small
Y24.-	Repair Microvascular NOC
F40.-	Repair Mouth NEC
T79.-	Repair Muscle
C37.4	Repair Muscle Eye NEC
H36.-	Repair Muscle Levator Ani
H36.1	Repair Muscle Pelvic Floor NEC
S66.2	Repair Nail Bed
E21.-	Repair Nasopharynx
A30.-	Repair Nerve Cranial
A62.-	Repair Nerve Peripheral Microsurgical
A62.-	Repair Nerve Peripheral Multiple Microsurgical
A64.-	Repair Nerve Peripheral NEC
Y26.-	Repair NOC
R32.-	Repair Obstetric Laceration
R32.-	Repair Obstetric Tear
F63.4	Repair Obturator
G23.-	Repair Oesophageal Hiatus
G07.-	Repair Oesophagus
C05.-	Repair Orbit Plastic
K09.4	Repair Ostium Primum Persistent
Q45.-	Repair Ovary
F29.-	Repair Palate Cleft
F29.-	Repair Palate Cleft Plastic
F30.-	Repair Palate NEC
F30.-	Repair Palate Plastic NEC
P23.5	Repair Paravaginal
H36.1	Repair Pelvic Floor Muscle NEC
N28.6	Repair Penis Fracture
K71.2	Repair Pericardium
R32.5	Repair Perineum Sphincter Mucosa Anus Obstetric Laceration
E21.-	Repair Pharynx
Y26.2	Repair Plastic NOC
G40.2	Repair Pylorus Atresia Congenital
G41.2	Repair Pylorus Perforation
E07.1	Repair Pyriform Aperture Stenosis
P25.3	Repair Rectovaginal Fistula
H42.6	Repair Rectum Prolapse Perineal NEC
T79.3	Repair Rotator Cuff Revisional
T79.-	Repair Rotator Cuff Shoulder Plastic
F48.3	Repair Salivary Gland NEC
C57.2	Repair Sclera
K13.-	Repair Septum Atrial Defect Transluminal Percutaneous
K09.-	Repair Septum Atrioventricular Defect
K12.-	Repair Septum Heart Defect NEC
K13.-	Repair Septum Heart Defect Transluminal
K10.-	Repair Septum Interatrial Defect NEC
K11.-	Repair Septum Interventricular Defect NEC
K13.-	Repair Septum Ventricular Defect Transluminal Percutaneous
T79.4	Repair Shoulder Rotator Cuff Multiple Tears Plastic

T79.5	Repair Shoulder Rotator Cuff Multiple Tears Revisional
K20.4	Repair Sinus Coronary Abnormality
E15.3	Repair Sinus Sphenoidal
V12.5	Repair Skull NEC
N18.-	Repair Spermatic Cord
J34.-	Repair Sphincter Oddi Plastic
A49.-	Repair Spina Bifida
J72.4	Repair Spleen
G36.-	Repair Stomach NEC
K37.3	Repair Subaortic Stenosis
K37.4	Repair Supra-aortic Stenosis
V21.8	Repair Temporomandibular Joint NEC
T67.-	Repair Tendon NEC
T67.-	Repair Tendon Primary
T68.-	Repair Tendon Secondary
N13.7	Repair Testis Rupture
K04.-	Repair Tetralogy Fallot
M22.-	Repair Ureter
M73.-	Repair Urethra
P25.2	Repair Urethrovaginal Fistula
P25.4	Repair Uterovaginal Fistula
P25.-	Repair Vagina NEC
P32.-	Repair Vagina Other Plastic
P21.-	Repair Vagina Plastic
P22.-	Repair Vagina Prolapse & Amputation Cervix Uteri
P23.-	Repair Vagina Prolapse NEC
P24.-	Repair Vagina Vault
K38.6	Repair Valsalva Aneurysm Aortic Sinus
K26.-	Repair Valve Aortic Plastic
K25.-	Repair Valve Mitral Plastic
K28.-	Repair Valve Pulmonary Plastic
K27.-	Repair Valve Tricuspid Plastic
K29.6	Repair Valve Truncal Plastic
L79.6	Repair Vein Caval Anomalous Connection
L80.1	Repair Vein Pulmonary Stenosis
L82.-	Repair Vein Valve
K24.4	Repair Ventricle Aneurysmal Left
K24.3	Repair Ventricle Aneurysmal Right
K08.-	Repair Ventricle Outlet Double
K24.2	Repair Ventricle Right Double Chambered
M37.2	Repair Vesicocolic Fistula
P25.1	Repair Vesicovaginal Fistula
P07.-	Repair Vulva
P07.-	Repair Vulva Skin
	Replacement – see also Autoreplacement
	Replacement – see also Prosthesis
	Replacement – see also Renewal
L18.-	Replacement Aorta Segment Aneurysmal Emergency
L19.-	Replacement Aorta Segment Aneurysmal NEC
L20.-	Replacement Aorta Segment Emergency NEC

L21.-	Replacement Aorta Segment NEC
K33.-	Replacement Aortic Root
K33.1	Replacement Aortic Root Autograft Valve Pulmonary
L29.1	Replacement Artery Carotid Graft
K42.-	Replacement Artery Coronary Allograft
K41.-	Replacement Artery Coronary Autograft NEC
K40.-	Replacement Artery Coronary Graft Vein Saphenous
K44.-	Replacement Artery Coronary NEC
K43.-	Replacement Artery Coronary Prosthetic
K44.2	Replacement Artery Coronary Revision
L56.-	Replacement Artery Femoral Aneurysmal Emergency
L57.-	Replacement Artery Femoral Aneurysmal NEC
L58.-	Replacement Artery Femoral Emergency NEC
L59.-	Replacement Artery Femoral NEC
L48.-	Replacement Artery Iliac Aneurysmal Emergency
L49.-	Replacement Artery Iliac Aneurysmal NEC
L50.-	Replacement Artery Iliac Emergency NEC
L51.-	Replacement Artery Iliac NEC
L56.-	Replacement Artery Popliteal Aneurysmal Emergency
L57.-	Replacement Artery Popliteal Aneurysmal NEC
L58.-	Replacement Artery Popliteal Emergency NEC
L59.-	Replacement Artery Popliteal NEC
W52.-	Replacement Bone Articulation Prosthetic Cemented NEC
W54.-	Replacement Bone Articulation Prosthetic NEC
W53.-	Replacement Bone Articulation Prosthetic Uncemented NEC
W05.-	Replacement Bone Prosthetic
C09.-	Replacement Canthal Tendon
K18.7	Replacement Conduit Cardiac Valved
C40.4	Replacement Conjunctiva Prosthetic
V01.2	Replacement Cranium Stored Bone Flap
V36.-	Replacement Disc Intervertebral Prosthetic
W46.-	Replacement Femur Head Prosthetic Cemented
W48.-	Replacement Femur Head Prosthetic NEC
W47.-	Replacement Femur Head Prosthetic Uncemented
K29.-	Replacement Heart Valve NEC
K30.-	Replacement Heart Valve Revision
W49.-	Replacement Humerus Head Prosthetic Cemented
W51.-	Replacement Humerus Head Prosthetic NEC
W50.-	Replacement Humerus Head Prosthetic Uncemented
O32.4	Replacement Joint Ankle Prosthetic Total Attention NEC (W)
O32.0	Replacement Joint Ankle Prosthetic Total Conversion From NEC (W)
O32.2	Replacement Joint Ankle Prosthetic Total Conversion To NEC (W)
O32.-	Replacement Joint Ankle Prosthetic Total NEC (W)
O32.5	Replacement Joint Ankle Prosthetic Total One Component Revision NEC (W)
O32.1	Replacement Joint Ankle Prosthetic Total Primary NEC (W)
O32.3	Replacement Joint Ankle Prosthetic Total Revision NEC (W)
O23.4	Replacement Joint Elbow Prosthetic Total Attention NEC (W)
O21.0	Replacement Joint Elbow Prosthetic Total Cemented Conversion From (W)
O21.2	Replacement Joint Elbow Prosthetic Total Cemented Conversion To (W)
O21.-	Replacement Joint Elbow Prosthetic Total Cemented NEC (W)

O21.1	Replacement Joint Elbow Prosthetic Total Cemented Primary (W)
O21.3	Replacement Joint Elbow Prosthetic Total Cemented Revision (W)
O23.0	Replacement Joint Elbow Prosthetic Total Conversion From NEC (W)
O23.2	Replacement Joint Elbow Prosthetic Total Conversion To NEC (W)
O23.-	Replacement Joint Elbow Prosthetic Total NEC (W)
O21.4	Replacement Joint Elbow Prosthetic Total One Component Cemented Revision (W)
O23.5	Replacement Joint Elbow Prosthetic Total One Component Revision NEC (W)
O22.4	Replacement Joint Elbow Prosthetic Total One Component Uncemented Revision (W)
O23.1	Replacement Joint Elbow Prosthetic Total Primary NEC (W)
O23.3	Replacement Joint Elbow Prosthetic Total Revision NEC (W)
O22.0	Replacement Joint Elbow Prosthetic Total Uncemented Conversion From (W)
O22.2	Replacement Joint Elbow Prosthetic Total Uncemented Conversion To (W)
O22.-	Replacement Joint Elbow Prosthetic Total Uncemented NEC (W)
O22.1	Replacement Joint Elbow Prosthetic Total Uncemented Primary (W)
O22.3	Replacement Joint Elbow Prosthetic Total Uncemented Revision (W)
W93.-	Replacement Joint Hip Hybrid Prosthetic Cemented Acetabular Component
W94.-	Replacement Joint Hip Hybrid Prosthetic Cemented Femoral Component
W95.-	Replacement Joint Hip Hybrid Prosthetic Cemented NEC
W37.-	Replacement Joint Hip Prosthetic Total Cemented
W39.-	Replacement Joint Hip Prosthetic Total NEC
W38.-	Replacement Joint Hip Prosthetic Total Uncemented
O18.-	Replacement Joint Knee Hybrid Prosthetic Cemented (W)
O18.4	Replacement Joint Knee Hybrid Prosthetic Cemented Attention (W)
O18.0	Replacement Joint Knee Hybrid Prosthetic Cemented Conversion From (W)
O18.2	Replacement Joint Knee Hybrid Prosthetic Cemented Conversion To (W)
O18.1	Replacement Joint Knee Hybrid Prosthetic Cemented Primary (W)
O18.3	Replacement Joint Knee Hybrid Prosthetic Cemented Revision (W)
W40.-	Replacement Joint Knee Prosthetic Total Cemented
W42.-	Replacement Joint Knee Prosthetic Total NEC
W41.-	Replacement Joint Knee Prosthetic Total Uncemented
W43.-	Replacement Joint Prosthetic Total Cemented NEC
W45.-	Replacement Joint Prosthetic Total NEC
W44.-	Replacement Joint Prosthetic Total Uncemented NEC
O07.-	Replacement Joint Shoulder Hybrid Prosthetic Cemented Glenoid Component (W)
O06.-	Replacement Joint Shoulder Hybrid Prosthetic Cemented Humeral Component (W)
O08.-	Replacement Joint Shoulder Hybrid Prosthetic Cemented NEC (W)
W96.-	Replacement Joint Shoulder Prosthetic Total Cemented
W98.-	Replacement Joint Shoulder Prosthetic Total NEC
W96.5	Replacement Joint Shoulder Prosthetic Total Reverse Polarity Cemented Primary
W96.6	Replacement Joint Shoulder Prosthetic Total Reverse Polarity Cemented Revision
W98.6	Replacement Joint Shoulder Prosthetic Total Reverse Polarity Primary NEC
W98.7	Replacement Joint Shoulder Prosthetic Total Reverse Polarity Revision NEC
W97.5	Replacement Joint Shoulder Prosthetic Total Reverse Polarity Uncemented Primary
W97.6	Replacement Joint Shoulder Prosthetic Total Reverse Polarity Uncemented Revision
W97.-	Replacement Joint Shoulder Prosthetic Total Uncemented
V20.-	Replacement Joint Temporomandibular Prosthetic
W72.-	Replacement Ligament Prosthetic
J01.3	Replacement Liver Transplant
E98.-	Replacement Nicotine Therapy
Y01.-	Replacement NOC

D16.-	Replacement Ossicular Chain
O26.4	Replacement Radius Head Prosthetic Attention NEC (W)
O24.-	Replacement Radius Head Prosthetic Cemented (W)
O24.0	Replacement Radius Head Prosthetic Cemented Conversion From (W)
O24.2	Replacement Radius Head Prosthetic Cemented Conversion To (W)
O24.1	Replacement Radius Head Prosthetic Cemented Primary (W)
O24.3	Replacement Radius Head Prosthetic Cemented Revision (W)
O26.0	Replacement Radius Head Prosthetic Conversion From NEC (W)
O26.2	Replacement Radius Head Prosthetic Conversion To NEC (W)
O26.-	Replacement Radius Head Prosthetic NEC (W)
O26.1	Replacement Radius Head Prosthetic Primary NEC (W)
O26.3	Replacement Radius Head Prosthetic Revision NEC (W)
O25.-	Replacement Radius Head Prosthetic Uncemented (W)
O25.0	Replacement Radius Head Prosthetic Uncemented Conversion From (W)
O25.2	Replacement Radius Head Prosthetic Uncemented Conversion To (W)
O25.1	Replacement Radius Head Prosthetic Uncemented Primary (W)
O25.3	Replacement Radius Head Prosthetic Uncemented Revision (W)
S52.6	Replacement Subcutaneous Tissue Hormone
C09.-	Replacement Tendon Canthus
	Replacement Testis – see also Placement Testis
N10.-	Replacement Testis Prosthetic
	Replacement Tube – see Tube
M21.-	Replacement Ureter NEC
M33.3	Replacement Ureteric Stent Metallic NEC
M33.4	Replacement Ureteric Stent Plastic NEC
Q12.2	Replacement Uterine Cavity Contraceptive Device
K26.-	Replacement Valve Aortic
K25.-	Replacement Valve Mitral
K28.-	Replacement Valve Pulmonary
K35.7	Replacement Valve Pulmonary Transluminal Percutaneous
K27.-	Replacement Valve Tricuspid
K29.7	Replacement Valve Truncal
L94.4	Replacement Vein Port Subcutaneous Transluminal Percutaneous
A73.6	Replantation & Transfer Nerve Peripheral
L45.2	Replantation Artery Coeliac
L45.2	Replantation Artery Mesenteric
L41.3	Replantation Artery Renal
L45.2	Replantation Artery Suprarenal
J27.1	Replantation Bile Duct Common Duodenum & Excision Ampulla Vater
Q30.2	Replantation Fallopian Tube
X02.-	Replantation Limb Lower
X01.-	Replantation Limb Upper
A57.6	Replantation Nerve Spinal Into Spinal Cord
Y04.-	Replantation NOC
X03.-	Replantation Organ NEC
Q45.1	Replantation Ovary
J69.1	Replantation Spleen Fragments & Excision Total
F08.3	Replantation Tooth
M20.-	Replantation Ureter
	Repositioning – see also Resiting

K06.-	Repositioning Arteries Great Transposed
F08.4	Repositioning Tooth
R30.1	Repositioning Uterus Delivered Inverted
R12.3	Repositioning Uterus Gravid Retroverted
K27.5	Repositioning Valve Tricuspid
L79.4	Repositioning Vena Cava Filter
A48.5	Reprogramming Spinal Cord Neurostimulator
	Resection – see also Excision
M42.1	Resection Bladder Lesion Endoscopic
M42.1	Resection Bladder Lesion Transurethral
M56.1	Resection Bladder Outlet Female Endoscopic
M55.1	Resection Bladder Outlet Female Open
M65.-	Resection Bladder Outlet Male Endoscopic
M64.1	Resection Bladder Outlet Male Open
H23.6	Resection Bowel Lower Lesion Sigmoidoscope Fibreoptic NEC
H23.1	Resection Bowel Lower Lesion Snare Sigmoidoscope Fibreoptic
H23.5	Resection Bowel Lower Lesion Submucosal Sigmoidoscope Fibreoptic
E48.1	Resection Bronchus Lesion Snare Endoscopic NEC
E50.1	Resection Bronchus Lesion Snare Endoscopic Rigid
E46.1	Resection Bronchus Sleeve & Anastomosis
H20.1	Resection Caecum Lesion Snare Endoscopic Fibreoptic
H20.1	Resection Caecum Lesion Snare Endoscopic NEC
E48.1	Resection Carina Lesion Snare Endoscopic NEC
E50.1	Resection Carina Lesion Snare Endoscopic Rigid
W82.-	Resection Cartilage Semilunar Endoscopic
H20.1	Resection Colon Lesion Snare Endoscopic Fibreoptic
H20.1	Resection Colon Lesion Snare Endoscopic NEC
H23.1	Resection Colon Lesion Snare Sigmoidoscope Fibreoptic
H20.5	Resection Colon Lesion Submucosal Endoscopic Fibreoptic
H26.7	Resection Colon Sigmoid Lesion Sigmoidoscope Rigid NEC
H23.1	Resection Colon Sigmoid Lesion Snare Endoscopic NEC
H23.1	Resection Colon Sigmoid Lesion Snare Sigmoidoscope Fibreoptic
H26.1	Resection Colon Sigmoid Lesion Snare Sigmoidoscope Rigid
H23.5	Resection Colon Sigmoid Lesion Submucosal Sigmoidoscope Fibreoptic
H26.6	Resection Colon Sigmoid Lesion Submucosal Sigmoidoscope Rigid
N22.5	Resection Duct Ejaculatory
G54.1	Resection Duodenum Lesion Snare NEC
G43.1	Resection Duodenum Prox. Lesion Snare & Exam. U.G.I. Tract Endoscopic Fibreoptic
G43.1	Resection Duodenum Prox. Lesion Snare & Exam. U.G.I. Tract Endoscopic NEC
C31.-	Resection Eye Muscle & Recession
C31.-	Resection Eye Muscle Bilateral
C33.-	Resection Eye Muscle NEC
G43.1	Resection Gastrointestinal Tract Upper Lesion Snare Endo. Fibreoptic
G43.1	Resection Gastrointestinal Tract Upper Lesion Snare Endoscopic NEC
G42.1	Resection Gastrointestinal Tract Upper Lesion Submucosal Endo. Fibreoptic
G42.1	Resection Gastrointestinal Tract Upper Lesion Submucosal Endoscopic NEC
K55.5	Resection Heart Tumour
H07.1	Resection Ileocaecal
G73.4	Resection Ileocolic Anastomosis
G73.3	Resection Ileostomy

M10.1	Resection Kidney Lesion Endoscopic
E34.-	Resection Larynx Lesion Endoscopic Microtherapeutic
J02.3	Resection Liver Section
J02.3	Resection Liver Segment
E48.1	Resection Lung Lesion Snare Endoscopic NEC
E50.1	Resection Lung Lesion Snare Endoscopic Rigid
C31.-	Resection Muscle Eye & Recession
C31.-	Resection Muscle Eye Bilateral
C33.-	Resection Muscle Eye NEC
G43.1	Resection Oesophagus Lesion Snare & Exam. U.G.I. Tract Endo. Fibreoptic
G43.1	Resection Oesophagus Lesion Snare & Exam. U.G.I. Tract Endoscopic NEC
G14.1	Resection Oesophagus Lesion Snare Endoscopic Fibreoptic
G14.1	Resection Oesophagus Lesion Snare Endoscopic NEC
G14.6	Resection Oesophagus Lesion Submucosal Endoscopic Fibreoptic
Y05.4	Resection Organ Ante Situm Hypothermic NOC
Y05.4	Resection Organ Ex Vivo NOC
T42.1	Resection Peritoneum Lesion Access Minimal
T42.1	Resection Peritoneum Lesion Endoscopic
M65.-	Resection Prostate Endoscopic
M65.-	Resection Prostate Transurethral
H33.-	Resection Rectum Anterior & Anastomosis
H23.1	Resection Rectum Lesion Snare Endoscopic NEC
H23.1	Resection Rectum Lesion Snare Sigmoidoscope Fibreoptic
H26.1	Resection Rectum Lesion Snare Sigmoidoscope Rigid
H23.5	Resection Rectum Lesion Submucosal Sigmoidoscope Fibreoptic
H26.6	Resection Rectum Lesion Submucosal Sigmoidoscope Rigid
H33.7	Resection Rectum Perineal
H41.2	Resection Rectum Tumour Peranal
H41.5	Resection Rectum Using Staples Peranal
E48.1	Resection Respiratory Tract Lower Lesion Snare Endoscopic NEC
E50.1	Resection Respiratory Tract Lower Lesion Snare Endoscopic Rigid
C53.1	Resection Sclera Punch
H26.6	Resection Sigmoid Colon Lesion Submucosal Sigmoidoscope Rigid
G43.1	Resection Stomach Lesion Snare Endoscopic Fibreoptic
G43.1	Resection Stomach Lesion Snare Endoscopic NEC
G17.1	Resection Stomach Lesion Snare Gastroscope Rigid
E48.1	Resection Trachea Lesion Snare Endoscopic NEC
E50.1	Resection Trachea Lesion Snare Endoscopic Rigid
M32.6	Resection Ureteric Orifice Transurethral Endoscopic
Q17.1	Resection Uterus Lesion Endoscopic
A12.5	Reservoir Cerebrospinal Fluid Subcutaneous Creation
V04.-	Reshaping Cranium
	Resiting – see also Repositioning
K60.2	Resiting Cardiac Pacemaker System Lead Intravenous
K61.2	Resiting Cardiac Pacemaker System Lead NEC
K59.3	Resiting Cardioverter Defibrillator Lead
K72.2	Resiting Cardioverter Defibrillator Lead Subcutaneous
H32.1	Resiting Colostomy
G75.6	Resiting Ileostomy
	Resiting Prosthesis – see Prosthesis site

Y15.4	Resiting Stent NOC
L91.3	Resiting Venous Catheter Central
E48.-	Respiratory Tract Lower Operations Endoscopic NEC
E50.-	Respiratory Tract Lower Operations Endoscopic Rigid
Z24.-	Respiratory Tract site NEC
E94.-	Response Bronchodilator
F13.-	Restoration Crown
F13.-	Restoration Tooth
	Resurfacing Arthroplasty – see Arthroplasty Joint Resurfacing
	Resurfacing Hemiarthroplasty Head of Humerus – see Hemiarthroplasty
X50.-	Resuscitation External
	Resuture – see also Suture
T28.3	Resuture Abdominal Wall
Y25.-	Resuture NOC
C80.-	Retina Membrane Operations NEC
C54.-	Retina Operations Buckling Attachment
C84.-	Retina Operations NEC
Z19.3	Retina site
C84.6	Retinectomy Relieving
C81.2	Retinopexy Laser for Detachment
C85.-	Retinopexy NEC
C84.6	Retinotomy NEC
V16.2	Retrusion Mandible & Osteotomy
K23.4	Revascularisation Heart NEC
K23.4	Revascularisation Heart Wall
L97.1	Revascularisation Impotence
	Reversal – see Primary Operation site
	Revision – see Operation Revision
	Revision – see Primary Operation
	Revision Anastomosis – see Anastomosis site
C65.3	Revision Bleb Following Glaucoma Surgery
	Revision Bypass – see Bypass site
	Revision Connection – see Connection site
H66.2	Revision Ileoanal Pouch
C65.3	Revision Iris Bleb
E11.4	Revision Nasal Prosthesis Fixtures Attachment
	Revision Neurolysis – see Neurolysis site
	Revision Prosthesis – see Prosthesis site
	Revision Reconstruction – see Reconstruction site
	Revision Release – see Release site
Y71.-	Revisional Operations NOC
E02.-	Rhinoplasty
E17.4	Rhinotomy Nasal Sinus Lateral NEC
A57.2	Rhizotomy Nerve Root Spinal
Z74.-	Rib Cage site NEC
Z74.-	Rib site
Z94.2	Right Sided Operations
Q36.-	Ringing Fallopian Tube Access Minimal NEC
Q35.3	Ringing Fallopian Tube Bilateral Access Minimal
Q35.3	Ringing Fallopian Tube Bilateral Endoscopic

Q27.2	Ringing Fallopian Tube Bilateral Open
Q36.-	Ringing Fallopian Tube Endoscopic NEC
Q28.-	Ringing Fallopian Tube Open NEC
F12.2	Root Canal Tooth Therapy
X23.6	Rotation Plasty Ankle Correction Leg Deformity Congenital Reversal
R14.1	Rupture Amniotic Membrane Forewater
R14.2	Rupture Amniotic Membrane Hindwater
M10.5	Rupture Kidney Pelviureteric Junction Stenosis Endoscopic Endoluminal Balloon
M27.6	Rupture Ureter Stenosis Ureteroscopic Endoluminal Balloon

S

Z11.-	Sacral Plexus site
A59.-	Sacrifice Nerve Peripheral
T65.1	Sacrifice Tendon
P24.2	Sacrocolpopexy
Q54.5	Sacrohysteropexy
Z75.-	Sacrum site
Z26.-	Salivary Apparatus site
F58.-	Salivary Duct Operations NEC
F53.-	Salivary Duct Operations Open NEC
Z26.7	Salivary Duct site
F48.-	Salivary Gland Operations NEC
Z26.4	Salivary Gland site
Q22.2	Salpingectomy Bilateral NEC
Q24.2	Salpingectomy NEC
Q25.-	Salpingectomy Partial
Q23.-	Salpingectomy Unilateral NEC
Q41.1	Salpingography
Q22.1	Salpingoophorectomy Bilateral
Q24.1	Salpingoophorectomy NEC
Q23.-	Salpingoophorectomy Unilateral
Q30.4	Salpingostomy
Q31.-	Salpingotomy
X36.4	Salvage Blood Autologous
X36.4	Salvage Cell Autologous Perioperative
X36.4	Salvage Cell Autologous Post-operative
H25.2	Sampling Bowel Lower Bacterial Overgrowth NEC
R10.-	Sampling Chorionic Villus NEC
R05.3	Sampling Chorionic Villus Percutaneous
R02.-	Sampling Fetal Blood Fetoscopic
R05.2	Sampling Fetal Blood Percutaneous
T86.-	Sampling Lymph Nodes
M30.3	Sampling Urine Ureteric Endoscopic
X36.3	Sampling Venous NEC
J77.1	Sampling Venous Portal Transhepatic Percutaneous
W18.2	Saucerisation Bone
F16.4	Scaling Tooth
	Scan – see also Imaging
R37.1	Scan Biophysical Profile
U14.-	Scan Bone Nuclear
U10.7	Scan Cardiac Multiple Gated Acquisition

R40.2	Scan Cervix Length
R36.1	Scan Dating
U13.1	Scan Dual Emission X-ray Absorptiometry
R37.5	Scan Fetal Ascites
R37.3	Scan Fetal Biometry
R37.3	Scan Growth NEC
U16.1	Scan Hepatobiliary Nuclear
R38.2	Scan Liquor Volume
U15.1	Scan Lung Perfusion NEC
U15.2	Scan Lung Ventilation NEC
T91.2	Scan Lymph Node Sentinel
U17.1	Scan Meckel's
R36.3	Scan Mid Trimester
U10.6	Scan Myocardial Perfusion
R37.4	Scan Nuchal Translucency
R37.-	Scan Obstetric Non-routine Fetal Observations
R38.-	Scan Obstetric Non-routine Other
R36.-	Scan Obstetric Routine
R38.1	Scan Placenta Localisation
R37.6	Scan Rhesus Detailed
R37.2	Scan Structural Detailed
U06.5	Scan Thyroid Gland
U15.3	Scan Ventilation Perfusion
R36.2	Scan Viability
U23.2	Scan White Cell Indium 111
U23.3	Scan White Cell Technetium 99
	Scanning – see Scan
Y90.3	Scanning NEC
Z72.2	Scaphoid site
U18.1	Scintimammography
C57.-	Sclera Operations NEC
Z18.3	Sclera site
C52.1	Sclerectomy Deep with Spacer
C52.2	Sclerectomy Deep Without Spacer
C54.1	Scleroplasty Overlay
G43.4	Sclerotherapy Gastrointestinal Tract Upper Lesion Endoscopic Fibreoptic
G43.4	Sclerotherapy Gastrointestinal Tract Upper Lesion Endoscopic NEC
H52.3	Sclerotherapy Haemorrhoid
N11.6	Sclerotherapy Hydrocele Sac Injection
L86.1	Sclerotherapy Leg Vein Varicose
L86.2	Sclerotherapy Leg Vein Varicose Foam Ultrasound Guided
Y12.1	Sclerotherapy Lesion NOC
G14.4	Sclerotherapy Oesophagus Varices Injection Endoscopic Fibreoptic
G14.4	Sclerotherapy Oesophagus Varices Injection Endoscopic NEC
G10.5	Sclerotherapy Oesophagus Varices Injection Open
G17.4	Sclerotherapy Stomach Varices Injection Gastroscope Rigid
C55.-	Sclerotomy
M17.1	Screening Kidney Live Donor
N03.-	Scrotum Operations NEC
Z43.1	Scrotum site

N03.-	Scrotum Skin Operations NEC
Z43.1	Scrotum Skin site
Y71.2	Secondary Operations NOC
C49.1	Section Cornea
Y84.2	Sedation NEC
C80.4	Segmentation Epiretinal Fibrovascular Membrane
D26.-	Semi-circular Canal Operations
N22.-	Seminal Vesicle Operations
Z43.5	Seminal Vesicle site
C67.1	Separation Ciliary Body
X25.4	Separation Tarsal Coalition
X17.-	Separation Twins Conjoined
K14.4	Septation Atrial Surgical
K14.3	Septectomy Atrial
E07.2	Septodermoplasty Nose
E03.6	Septoplasty Nose NEC
E07.3	Septorhinoplasty NEC
E02.4	Septorhinoplasty Using Graft
E02.3	Septorhinoplasty Using Implant
K15.2	Septostomy Atrial Closed
K14.2	Septostomy Atrial NEC
K16.-	Septostomy Atrial Transluminal Percutaneous
W18.3	Sequestrectomy Bone
U08.4	Series Gastrointestinal Upper Imaging
H55.4	Seton Anal Fistula High Insertion & Laying Open Track Partial HFQ
X16.-	Sex Development Disorders Operations
X15.-	Sexual Transformation Operations
B36.-	Sharing Nipple
F06.3	Shave Lip
F06.3	Shave Lip Mucosa
F06.3	Shave Lip Skin
E09.4	Shave Nose Skin
W83.3	Shaving Cartilage Articular Endoscopic
C84.4	Sheathotomy Retinal Vascular
X12.3	Shortening Amputation Stump
W17.4	Shortening Bone
T70.-	Shortening Tendon
Q52.3	Shortening Uterus Ligament Broad
	Shunt – see also Anastomosis
	Shunt – see also Connection
L06.-	Shunt Aortopulmonary NEC
L05.-	Shunt Aortopulmonary Prosthesis Interposition Tube Creation
L74.-	Shunt Arteriovenous
L08.-	Shunt Artery Subclavian Pulmonary NEC
L07.-	Shunt Artery Subclavian Pulmonary Prosthesis Tube Creation
A14.-	Shunt Cerebroventricular Attention NEC
A13.-	Shunt Cerebroventricular Catheter Maintenance
A13.-	Shunt Cerebroventricular Component Attention
A12.1	Shunt Cerebroventricular Creation
A14.4	Shunt Cerebroventricular Irrigation

A14.-	Shunt Cerebroventricular NEC
A14.3	Shunt Cerebroventricular Removal
R04.-	Shunt Fetal Insertion Percutaneous
A53.6	Shunt Lumbar Subcutaneous
A53.-	Shunt Lumboperitoneal
L77.-	Shunt Mesocaval
L81.-	Shunt Peritoneovenous
L81.-	Shunt Peritovenous
L77.-	Shunt Portocaval
L77.-	Shunt Portosystemic
J11.4	Shunt Portosystemic Intrahepatic Transjugular
A53.8	Shunt Spinal Attention
L77.-	Shunt Splenorenal
A53.-	Shunt Syringoperitoneal
A53.-	Shunt Thecoperitoneal
A13.-	Shunt Ventricle Brain Catheter Maintenance
A12.-	Shunt Ventricle Brain Creation
A14.-	Shunt Ventricle Brain Removal
A12.2	Shunt Ventriculoatrial Creation
A13.-	Shunt Ventriculoperitoneal Catheter Maintenance
A12.4	Shunt Ventriculoperitoneal Creation
A14.-	Shunt Ventriculoperitoneal Removal
A13.-	Shunt Ventriculopleural Catheter Maintenance
A12.3	Shunt Ventriculopleural Creation
A14.-	Shunt Ventriculopleural Removal
A13.-	Shunt Ventriculovascular Catheter Maintenance
A12.2	Shunt Ventriculovascular Creation
A14.-	Shunt Ventriculovascular Removal
F48.4	Sialography
H25.-	Sigmoidoscopy Fibreoptic
H25.-	Sigmoidoscopy NEC
H28.-	Sigmoidoscopy Rigid
Y39.1	Sinogram NOC
H60.4	Sinography Pilonidal Abscess
H60.4	Sinography Pilonidal Cyst
H60.4	Sinography Pilonidal Sinus
Z50.7	Skin Ankle site
Z50.1	Skin Arm site
Z49.2	Skin Axilla site
Z49.1	Skin Breast site
Z49.5	Skin Buttock site
	Skin Ear External – see also Ear External Skin
D06.-	Skin Ear External Operations NEC
Z20.1	Skin Ear External site
	Skin Eyebrow – see also Eyebrow
C10.-	Skin Eyebrow Operations
Z16.2	Skin Eyebrow site
	Skin Eyelid – see also Eyelid Skin
C22.-	Skin Eyelid Operations NEC
Z16.4	Skin Eyelid site

Z47.-	Skin Face site
Z50.3	Skin Finger site
	Skin Flap – see Flap site
Z50.5	Skin Foot site
Z49.7	Skin Groin site
Z50.2	Skin Hand site
Z48.-	Skin Head site NEC
Z50.4	Skin Leg site
	Skin Lip – see also Lip
F06.-	Skin Lip Operations NEC
Z25.1	Skin Lip site
Z48.2	Skin Neck site
	Skin Nipple – see also Nipple
B35.-	Skin Nipple Operations
Z15.6	Skin Nipple site
	Skin Nose External – see also Nose External Skin
E09.-	Skin Nose External Operations
Z22.-	Skin Nose External site
S60.-	Skin Operations NEC
	Skin Penis – see also Penis Skin
N32.-	Skin Penis Operations NEC
Z42.7	Skin Penis site
	Skin Perineum Female – see also Perineum Skin Female
P13.-	Skin Perineum Female Operations NEC
Z44.4	Skin Perineum Female site
	Skin Perineum Male – see also Perineum Skin Male
N24.-	Skin Perineum Male Operations
Z43.6	Skin Perineum Male site
N30.-	Skin Prepuce Operations
Z42.6	Skin Prepuce site
	Skin Scrotum – see also Scrotum Skin
N03.-	Skin Scrotum Operations NEC
Z43.1	Skin Scrotum site
Z49.6	Skin Shoulder site
Z50.-	Skin site NEC
U27.-	Skin Test Application Diagnostic
U28.-	Skin Test Diagnostic NEC
Z50.6	Skin Toe site
Z49.-	Skin Trunk site
	Skin Umbilicus – see Umbilicus Skin
Z53.2	Skin Umbilicus site
	Skin Vulva – see also Vulva Skin
P09.-	Skin Vulva Operations NEC
Z44.3	Skin Vulva site
H42.3	Sling Supralevator Insertion
M52.1	Sling Suprapubic
N30.-	Slit Prepuce
Q55.-	Smear Cervical
F43.1	Smear Mucosa Buccal
Q55.-	Smear Papanicolau

	Snare Removal – see Resection site
W79.-	Soft Tissue Operations Joint Toe
T96.-	Soft Tissue Operations NEC
Z62.-	Soft Tissue site NEC
N20.-	Spermatic Cord Operations NEC
Z43.4	Spermatic Cord site
E15.-	Sphenoid Sinus Operations NEC
Z23.4	Sphenoid Sinus site
J39.-	Sphincter Oddi Operations Endoscopic Therapeutic NEC
J36.-	Sphincter Oddi Operations NEC
Z30.5	Sphincter Oddi site
J34.-	Sphincteroplasty Bile Duct Approach Duodenal
J34.-	Sphincteroplasty Pancreatic Duct Approach Duodenal
J34.-	Sphincteroplasty Papilla Vater
J39.1	Sphincterotomy Ampulla Vater Accessory Endoscopic
H56.2	Sphincterotomy Anus Lateral
J35.-	Sphincterotomy Bile Duct Approach Duodenal
M66.1	Sphincterotomy Bladder Sphincter External Male Endoscopic
H51.2	Sphincterotomy Haemorrhoid Internal Partial
J35.-	Sphincterotomy Pancreatic Duct Approach Duodenal
J35.-	Sphincterotomy Papilla Vater
J38.-	Sphincterotomy Papilla Vater Endoscopic
J38.-	Sphincterotomy Sphincter Oddi Endoscopic
A51.-	Spinal Cord Meninges Operations NEC
Z06.4	Spinal Cord Meninges site
A48.-	Spinal Cord Operations NEC
A45.-	Spinal Cord Operations Open NEC
Z06.-	Spinal Cord site
Z07.-	Spinal Nerve Root site
A45.-	Spinal Tract Operations Open NEC
Y48.-	Spine Approach Back
Y48.-	Spine Approach Laminectomy
Y50.1	Spine Approach Transperitoneal
Y49.2	Spine Approach Transthoracic
V55.-	Spine Levels
V54.-	Spine Operations NEC
O16.2	Spine site NEC (Z)
E93.2	Spirometry
J72.-	Spleen Operations NEC
Z31.3	Spleen site
J69.-	Splenectomy NEC
J70.1	Splenectomy Partial
O30.2	Splenic Flexure site (Z)
X49.-	Splint
F63.5	Splinting Teeth
V18.4	Spring Skull Attention
V18.2	Spring Skull Insertion
V18.6	Spring Skull Removal
O27.-	Stabilisation Joint Glenohumeral (W)
O27.2	Stabilisation Joint Glenohumeral Repair Capsule Labrum Anterior & Posterior (W)

O27.3	Stabilisation Joint Glenohumeral Repair Capsule Labrum Anterior (W)
O27.4	Stabilisation Joint Glenohumeral Repair Capsule Labrum Posterior (W)
W77.-	Stabilisation Joint NEC
V40.-	Stabilisation Spine
V40.1	Stabilisation Spine Non-rigid
Y70.3	Staged Operations First NOC
Y71.1	Staged Operations Subsequent NOC
G45.4	Staining Stomach Mucosa NEC
D17.-	Stapedectomy
W27.-	Stapling Epiphysis
Y26.3	Stapling NOC
G30.4	Stapling Stomach
Y99.-	Status Donor
A81.1	Stellate Ganglion Blockade
	Stent – see Operation site Stent
	Stent Graft Insertion – see Insertion site Stent Graft
	Stent Implantation – see Implantation site Stent
S54.6	Sterilisation & Cleansing Skin Burnt Head
S55.6	Sterilisation & Cleansing Skin Burnt NEC
S54.6	Sterilisation & Cleansing Skin Burnt Neck
S56.6	Sterilisation & Cleansing Skin Head
S57.6	Sterilisation & Cleansing Skin NEC
S56.6	Sterilisation & Cleansing Skin Neck
	Sterilisation Female – see also Operation
Q37.-	Sterilisation Female Reversal Endoscopic
Q29.-	Sterilisation Female Reversal Open
	Sterilisation Male – see Operation
Y49.1	Sternotomy Median Approach
T03.1	Sternotomy Median Exploratory
Z74.-	Sternum site
	Stimulation Nerve – see Neurostimulator
W33.-	Stimulator Bone Electromagnetic
Y90.1	Stimulator Nerve Electrical Transcutaneous Application
G44.-	Stomach Operations Endoscopic Fibreoptic NEC
G44.-	Stomach Operations Endoscopic Therapeutic NEC
G18.-	Stomach Operations Gastroscope Rigid NEC
G48.-	Stomach Operations NEC
G38.-	Stomach Operations Open NEC
G30.-	Stomach Operations Plastic
Z27.2	Stomach site
G35.-	Stomach Ulcer Operations
Q56.8	Storage Oocyte
U11.5	Stress Test Thallium
H54.1	Stretching Anorectal
P15.5	Stretching Hymen
C64.6	Stretching Iris
T83.3	Stretching Muscle
Y40.2	Stretching NOC
N30.5	Stretching Prepuce
G78.2	Strictureplasty Ileum

G78.2	Strictureplasty Intestine Small NEC
C09.2	Strip Periosteal Lateral
C09.3	Strip Periosteal Medial
C09.1	Strip Tarsal Lateral
L92.1	Stripping Catheter
T57.4	Stripping Fascia
L87.-	Stripping Leg Vein Varicose
W04.4	Stripping Muscle Os Calcis
M47.4	Studies Urodynamic Catheter Urethral
M48.2	Studies Urodynamic Tube Suprapubic
E93.3	Study Airways Resistance Body Plethysmographic
E93.4	Study Airways Resistance Forced Oscillation Technique
E92.3	Study Alveolar Carbon Monoxide
E94.-	Study Bronchial Reaction
E93.7	Study Expiratory & Inspiratory Flow Volume Loop
E93.1	Study Expiratory Peak Flow Rate
U23.4	Study Ferrokinetic
K58.-	Study Heart Conducting System
E93.7	Study Inspiratory & Expiratory Flow Volume Loop
E93.5	Study Lung Static Volume
A84.3	Study Nerve Conduction
R42.-	Study Obstetric Doppler
E91.3	Study Oxygen Desaturation Index
E93.6	Study Respiratory Muscle Strength
E93.-	Study Respiratory NEC
U17.2	Study Selenium 75 Homocholic Acid Taurine
A84.7	Study Sleep NEC
M12.-	Study Urinary Tract Upper Percutaneous
A22.-	Subarachnoid Space Operations
Z49.2	Subcutaneous Tissue Axilla site
Z49.1	Subcutaneous Tissue Breast site
Z49.5	Subcutaneous Tissue Buttock site
Z47.-	Subcutaneous Tissue Face site
Z48.-	Subcutaneous Tissue Head site NEC
Z48.2	Subcutaneous Tissue Neck site
S63.-	Subcutaneous Tissue Operations
S62.-	Subcutaneous Tissue Operations Other NEC
Z50.-	Subcutaneous Tissue site NEC
Z49.-	Subcutaneous Tissue Trunk site
Z26.3	Sublingual Gland site
F58.2	Submandibular Duct Operations NEC
F53.2	Submandibular Duct Operations Open NEC
Z26.6	Submandibular Duct site
Z26.2	Submandibular Gland site
	Suction Clearance – see Clearance
X58.-	Support Body System Artificial
X49.-	Support Bone Fracture External NEC
X49.-	Support Limb External NEC
E87.1	Support Oxygen Home
Y92.-	Support Radiotherapy

E89.-	Support Respiratory Other
E95.-	Support Tuberculosis
E85.-	Support Ventilation
Y73.3	Support Ventilatory
M52.1	Suprapubic Operation Sling
M49.8	Suprapubic Tube Operation Through
M51.2	Suspension Bladder Neck Endoscopic
M52.2	Suspension Bladder Neck Retropubic
M51.1	Suspension Urethra Abdominoperineal
M51.1	Suspension Urethra Abdominovaginal
Q54.4	Suspension Uterus Mesh NEC
Q54.1	Suspension Uterus NEC
P24.-	Suspension Vagina
	Suture – see also Resuture
T28.-	Suture Abdomen
T28.-	Suture Abdominal Wall
Q01.2	Suture Cervix Uteri & Excision
T05.-	Suture Chest Wall
C40.5	Suture Conjunctiva
C47.-	Suture Cornea
Q45.4	Suture Corpus Luteum Rupture
T16.5	Suture Diaphragm NEC
G52.-	Suture Duodenum Ulcer
	Suture Encirclement – see Cerclage
C35.3	Suture Eye Muscle Adjustable Insertion
C86.3	Suture Eye NEC
C10.4	Suture Eyebrow
C17.1	Suture Eyelid
C20.-	Suture Eyelid Protective
C17.1	Suture Eyelid Skin
Q30.5	Suture Fallopian Tube
F20.5	Suture Gingiva
C65.4	Suture Glaucoma Surgery Removal
F05.3	Suture Lip
F05.4	Suture Lip Removal
C65.5	Suture Lysis Eye Glaucoma Surgery Laser
F40.4	Suture Mouth NEC
C35.3	Suture Muscle Eye Adjustable Insertion
Y25.-	Suture NOC
E09.3	Suture Nose External
E09.3	Suture Nose External Skin
Q45.3	Suture Ovary
F30.7	Suture Palate
H42.-	Suture Perianal Sphincter Insertion
H42.-	Suture Perianal Sphincter Removal
W33.3	Suture Periosteum
C57.4	Suture Sclera
N03.3	Suture Scrotum
N03.3	Suture Scrotum Skin
S41.-	Suture Skin Head

S42.-	Suture Skin NEC
S41.-	Suture Skin Neck
S43.-	Suture Skin Removal
G35.-	Suture Stomach Ulcer
S41.-	Suture Subcutaneous Tissue Head
S42.-	Suture Subcutaneous Tissue NEC
S41.-	Suture Subcutaneous Tissue Neck
S43.-	Suture Subcutaneous Tissue Removal
F26.5	Suture Tongue
M22.1	Suture Ureter
P25.5	Suture Vagina
N18.2	Suture Vas Deferens NEC
	Suture Wound – see Suture Skin
Q55.6	Swab Genital Female
K06.1	Switch Arterial
K06.4	Switch Arterial Double
G71.7	Switch Duodenal Reversal
G71.6	Switch Duodenum
G28.4	Switch Duodenum & Sleeve Gastrectomy
A76.-	Sympathectomy Chemical
A75.-	Sympathectomy NEC
W79.3	Syndactylisation Toe Lesser
W69.-	Synovectomy
	Syringing – see Irrigation
A53.1	Syringostomy Cerebrospinal
K60.-	System Cardiac Pacemaker Intravenous
K61.-	System Cardiac Pacemaker NEC
K56.-	System Heart Assist Transluminal

T

L06.7	Takedown Anastomosis Aortopulmonary
K17.6	Takedown Cavopulmonary Connection Total
Z79.-	Talus site
C79.-	Tamponade Retina Operations
N11.5	Tapping Hydrocele Sac
T46.2	Tapping Peritoneum Ascites NEC
T46.9	Tapping Peritoneum NEC
X25.2	Tarsectomy Wedge Correction Foot Deformity Congenital
C18.5	Tarsomullerectomy
C16.-	Tarsorrhaphy
Z79.-	Tarsus site
C51.4	Tattooing Cornea
B36.4	Tattooing Nipple
Y39.5	Tattooing NOC
S60.3	Tattooing Skin
U22.1	Telemetry Electroencephalograph
X51.-	Temperature Change
Y70.5	Temporary Operations
T74.-	Tendon Operations NEC
T72.-	Tendon Sheath Operations NEC
	Tendon site – see Muscle site
T64.5	Tenodesis
T69.1	Tenolysis Primary
T69.2	Tenolysis Revision
T71.1	Tenosynovectomy
C34.-	Tenotomy Eye Muscle
C34.-	Tenotomy Muscle Eye
T70.-	Tenotomy NEC
	Terminalisation – see Amputation
	Termination Pregnancy – see Operation
U29.5	Test Adrenal Suppression
U29.6	Test Arginine Vasopressin Response Hypertonic Saline
U32.-	Test Blood Diagnostic
U32.1	Test Blood Human Immunodeficiency Virus
U25.-	Test Breath
E92.1	Test Carbon Monoxide Transfer
U34.1	Test Cardiac Provocation
U30.2	Test Carotid Sinus Massage
E92.5	Test Cycle Progressive with Measure of Gas Exchange
U29.4	Test Deprivation Water

U33.-	Test Diagnostic Other
U22.7	Test Executive Function Neuropsychology
U26.1	Test Glomerular Filtration Rate
U29.3	Test Glucose Tolerance
E95.1	Test Heaf
U29.2	Test Insulin Secretion Glucagon
U22.3	Test Intelligence Neuropsychology
E92.5	Test Jones Stage 2-4
U22.4	Test Language Neuropsychology
E92.-	Test Lung Function Exercise
E92.5	Test Lung Function Exercise Complex
E92.6	Test Lung Function Exercise Simple
E95.5	Test Mantoux
U22.5	Test Memory Neuropsychology
U22.-	Test Neuropsychology
U31.1	Test Pacemaker Distant
U22.6	Test Perception Neuropsychology
U29.1	Test Pituitary Anterior Function Insulin Stress
E92.-	Test Respiratory
U26.5	Test Schilling
U29.7	Test Short Synacthen
U27.-	Test Skin Application Diagnostic
U40.-	Test Skin Diagnostic
U28.-	Test Skin Diagnostic Other
U28.-	Test Skin for Urticaria NEC
U28.-	Test Skin Passive Transfer for Urticaria
U28.-	Test Skin Reverse Passive Transfer for Urticaria
U28.6	Test Skin Serum Autologous for Urticaria
U40.2	Test Skin Ultraviolet Diagnostic
E92.5	Test Treadmill Progressive with Measure of Gas Exchange
E92.2	Test Ventilation Distribution
U30.-	Testing Cardiovascular Autonomic
E91.-	Testing Oximetry
U31.-	Testing Pacemaker
U30.1	Testing Table Tilt
N13.-	Testis Operations NEC
Z43.2	Testis site
N13.2	Tether Testis
X37.1	Therapy Calcitonin Intramuscular
X66.-	Therapy Cognitive Behavioural
X61.-	Therapy Complementary
X65.7	Therapy Delivery Radionuclide NEC
A83.-	Therapy Electroconvulsive
X61.1	Therapy Functional Session
X37.2	Therapy Gold Intramuscular
X52.1	Therapy Hyperbaric
X51.1	Therapy Hypothermia
E97.1	Therapy Inhalation
E05.4	Therapy Internal Nose Laser
S58.-	Therapy Larvae

Y08.-	Therapy Laser NOC
S59.-	Therapy Leech
S59.2	Therapy Leech Skin
S59.1	Therapy Leech Skin Head
S59.1	Therapy Leech Skin Neck
X61.4	Therapy Movement NEC
E89.3	Therapy Nebuliser
E98.-	Therapy Nicotine Replacement
E87.2	Therapy Oxygen Long-term
	Therapy Photodynamic – see Photodynamic Therapy
X65.5	Therapy Radioactive Iodine Oral
X61.2	Therapy Relaxation Session
S12.-	Therapy Skin Light Ultraviolet
E98.-	Therapy Smoking Cessation
E95.3	Therapy Tuberculosis Directly Observed
V62.-	Thermocoagulation Disc Intervertebral Radiofrequency Percutaneous NEC
V62.-	Thermocoagulation Disc Intervertebral Radiofrequency Percutaneous Primary
V63.-	Thermocoagulation Disc Intervertebral Radiofrequency Percutaneous Revisional
U35.1	Thermography Blood Flow
U01.3	Thermography Body Whole
U18.2	Thermography Breast
U36.1	Thermography NEC
C88.1	Thermotherapy Retina Lesion Transpupillary
C88.1	Thermotherapy Subretina Lesion Transpupillary
S03.2	Thigh Lift
Y49.-	Thoracic Cavity Approach
T12.3	Thoracocentesis
T01.1	Thoracoplasty
	Thoracoscopic – refer to Index Introduction
Y74.-	Thoracoscopic Operations NEC
T11.-	Thoracoscopy
Y49.3	Thoracotomy Approach NEC
T03.-	Thoracotomy Exploratory
L25.3	Thrombectomy Aorta Bifurcation NEC
L26.3	Thrombectomy Aorta Bifurcation Transluminal Percutaneous
L74.5	Thrombectomy Arteriovenous Fistula
L38.3	Thrombectomy Artery Axillary NEC
L39.2	Thrombectomy Artery Axillary Transluminal Percutaneous
L38.3	Thrombectomy Artery Brachial NEC
L39.2	Thrombectomy Artery Brachial Transluminal Percutaneous
L30.3	Thrombectomy Artery Carotid NEC
L34.3	Thrombectomy Artery Cerebral NEC
L34.3	Thrombectomy Artery Circle Willis NEC
L46.1	Thrombectomy Artery Coeliac NEC
L62.2	Thrombectomy Artery Femoral NEC
L63.2	Thrombectomy Artery Femoral Transluminal Percutaneous
L53.2	Thrombectomy Artery Iliac NEC
L54.2	Thrombectomy Artery Iliac Transluminal Percutaneous
L46.1	Thrombectomy Artery Mesenteric NEC
L70.1	Thrombectomy Artery NEC

L62.2	Thrombectomy Artery Popliteal NEC
L63.2	Thrombectomy Artery Popliteal Transluminal Percutaneous
L12.4	Thrombectomy Artery Pulmonary NEC
L13.1	Thrombectomy Artery Pulmonary Transluminal Percutaneous
L42.1	Thrombectomy Artery Renal NEC
L43.2	Thrombectomy Artery Renal Transluminal Percutaneous
L38.3	Thrombectomy Artery Subclavian NEC
L39.2	Thrombectomy Artery Subclavian Transluminal Percutaneous
L46.1	Thrombectomy Artery Suprarenal NEC
L71.2	Thrombectomy Artery Transluminal Percutaneous
L38.3	Thrombectomy Artery Vertebral NEC
L39.2	Thrombectomy Artery Vertebral Transluminal Percutaneous
J10.5	Thrombectomy Blood Vessel Liver Transluminal Percutaneous NEC
J10.5	Thrombectomy Vein Hepatic Transluminal Percutaneous
L90.-	Thrombectomy Vein Open
J11.2	Thrombectomy Vein Portal Intrahepatic Transjugular
J10.5	Thrombectomy Vein Portal Transluminal Percutaneous
L96.2	Thromboembolectomy Aspiration Percutaneous
L96.1	Thromboembolectomy Mechanical Percutaneous
L04.1	Thromboendarterectomy Artery Pulmonary
L66.1	Thrombolysis Arterial Reconstruction Transluminal Percutaneous
L66.1	Thrombolysis Artery & Placement Stent Transluminal Percutaneous
K50.2	Thrombolysis Artery Coronary Transluminal Percutaneous Streptokinase
L71.6	Thrombolysis Artery Transluminal Percutaneous
L71.6	Thrombolysis Artery Transluminal Percutaneous Streptokinase
J10.6	Thrombolysis Blood Vessel Liver Transluminal Percutaneous NEC
L99.3	Thrombolysis Vein & Placement Stent Transluminal Percutaneous
L99.3	Thrombolysis Vein Angioplasty Transluminal Percutaneous
J10.6	Thrombolysis Vein Hepatic Transluminal Percutaneous
J11.3	Thrombolysis Vein Portal Intrahepatic Transjugular
J10.6	Thrombolysis Vein Portal Transluminal Percutaneous
L99.3	Thrombolysis Venous Reconstruction Transluminal Percutaneous
L99.4	Thrombolysis Venous Transluminal Percutaneous NEC
B18.-	Thymectomy
B20.-	Thymus Operations NEC
Z14.3	Thymus site
Z13.3	Thyroglossal Cyst site
B10.-	Thyroglossal Tissue Operations
Z13.4	Thyroglossal Tract site
B12.-	Thyroid Operations NEC
Z13.1	Thyroid site
B09.-	Thyroid Tissue Aberrant Operations
Z13.2	Thyroid Tissue Aberrant site
B08.-	Thyroidectomy
	Thyroplasty – see Medialisation Vocal Cord
Z78.1	Tibia & Fibula Shaft Combination site
Z77.-	Tibia site NEC
	Tissue Expander – see Expander Skin
	Toilet – see also Debridement
S54.-	Toilet Skin Burnt Head NEC

S55.-	Toilet Skin Burnt NEC
S54.-	Toilet Skin Burnt Neck NEC
S56.-	Toilet Skin Head NEC
S57.-	Toilet Skin NEC
S56.-	Toilet Skin Neck NEC
S54.-	Toilet Subcutaneous Tissue Burnt Head NEC
S55.-	Toilet Subcutaneous Tissue Burnt NEC
S54.-	Toilet Subcutaneous Tissue Burnt Neck NEC
S56.-	Toilet Subcutaneous Tissue Head NEC
S57.-	Toilet Subcutaneous Tissue NEC
S56.-	Toilet Subcutaneous Tissue Neck NEC
P27.2	Toilet Vagina
U08.1	Tomography Abdomen Computed NEC
U35.4	Tomography Arteries Pulmonary Computed
U01.1	Tomography Body Whole Computed
U13.6	Tomography Bone Computed
U05.1	Tomography Brain Computed
U10.1	Tomography Cardiac Calcium Scoring
U10.2	Tomography Cardiac Computed Angiography
U11.4	Tomography Cerebral Vessels Computed
U07.1	Tomography Chest Computed
U17.5	Tomography Colon Computed
U05.1	Tomography Head Computed
U13.6	Tomography Joint Computed
U37.2	Tomography Kidneys Computed
U10.4	Tomography Myocardial Positron Emission
U09.1	Tomography Pelvis Computed
U21.3	Tomography Positron Emission
U36.2	Tomography Positron Emission Computed Tomography
C87.3	Tomography Retina Computed
U21.4	Tomography Single Photon Emission Computed
U36.3	Tomography Single Photon Emission Computed Tomography
U06.1	Tomography Sinuses Computed
U05.4	Tomography Spinal Cord Computed
U05.4	Tomography Spine Computed
F26.-	Tongue Operations NEC
Z25.5	Tongue site
F36.-	Tonsil Operations NEC
Z25.7	Tonsil site
F34.-	Tonsillectomy
F34.7	Tonsillectomy Coblation Bilateral
F12.-	Tooth Apex Surgery
F17.-	Tooth Bridge Operations
F17.-	Tooth Crown Operations
F16.-	Tooth Operations NEC
F12.2	Tooth Root Canal Therapy
Z25.3	Tooth site NEC
Z25.2	Tooth Wisdom site
C60.1	Trabeculectomy
C61.1	Trabeculoplasty Laser

C61.2	Trabeculotomy
E48.-	Trachea Operations Endoscopic NEC
E50.-	Trachea Operations Endoscopic Rigid
E52.-	Trachea Operations NEC
E43.-	Trachea Operations Open NEC
E40.-	Trachea Operations Plastic
Z24.3	Trachea site
E49.-	Tracheobronchoscopy NEC
E43.3	Tracheopexy
E43.2	Tracheorrhaphy
E49.9	Tracheoscopy NEC
E42.-	Tracheostomy
Y52.1	Tracheostomy Approach
E42.3	Tracheotomy
W29.-	Traction Bone Skeletal
X49.4	Traction Skin
V50.1	Traction Skull Halo Ring & Jacket
V46.4	Traction Skull Skeletal Fracture Spine
K48.1	Transection Artery Coronary Muscle Bridge
M43.1	Transection Bladder Endoscopic
M41.3	Transection Bladder Open
A28.8	Transection Nerve Abducens (vi) Extracranial
A25.2	Transection Nerve Abducens (vi) NEC
A25.8	Transection Nerve Accessory (xi) Intracranial
A28.2	Transection Nerve Accessory (xi) NEC
A28.8	Transection Nerve Acoustic (viii) Extracranial
A25.5	Transection Nerve Acoustic (viii) NEC
A28.-	Transection Nerve Cranial Extracranial
A25.-	Transection Nerve Cranial Intracranial
A25.4	Transection Nerve Facial (vii) Intracranial
A28.8	Transection Nerve Facial (vii) NEC
A28.8	Transection Nerve Glossopharyngeal (ix) Extracranial
A25.6	Transection Nerve Glossopharyngeal (ix) NEC
A28.8	Transection Nerve Hypoglossal (xii) Extracranial
A25.8	Transection Nerve Hypoglossal (xii) NEC
A28.8	Transection Nerve Oculomotor (iii) Extracranial
A25.2	Transection Nerve Oculomotor (iii) NEC
A28.8	Transection Nerve Optic (ii) Extracranial
A25.1	Transection Nerve Optic (ii) NEC
A60.3	Transection Nerve Peripheral
A25.3	Transection Nerve Trigeminal (v) Intracranial
A28.1	Transection Nerve Trigeminal (v) NEC
A28.8	Transection Nerve Trochlear (iv) Extracranial
A25.2	Transection Nerve Trochlear (iv) NEC
A25.7	Transection Nerve Vagus (x) Intracranial
A27.-	Transection Nerve Vagus (x) NEC
G10.-	Transection Oesophagus
A07.5	Transections Subpial Multiple
A73.6	Transfer & Reimplantation Nerve Peripheral
Q13.-	Transfer Embryo

T50.1	Transfer Fascial Tissue
Q38.3	Transfer Gametes Intrafallopian Access Minimal
Q38.3	Transfer Gametes Intrafallopian Endoscopic
T76.1	Transfer Muscle Flap Free Tissue Microvascular
A62.-	Transfer Nerve Peripheral Microsurgical
W83.7	Transfer Osteochondral Endoscopic
T64.-	Transfer Tendon
W03.-	Transfer Tendon Extensor Hallucis Longus
N08.1	Transfer Testis Scrotum Microvascular Bilateral
N09.1	Transfer Testis Scrotum Microvascular Unilateral
W01.5	Transfer Thumb Opposition
W01.1	Transfer Toe Thumb Microvascular
Q21.1	Transfer Uterus Transmyometrial Embryo
X15.-	Transformation Sexual Operations
X32.-	Transfusion Blood Exchange
X32.1	Transfusion Blood Exchange Neonatal
X34.4	Transfusion Blood Expander
R01.1	Transfusion Blood Fetus Fetoscopic
R04.3	Transfusion Blood Fetus Percutaneous
X33.1	Transfusion Blood Intra-arterial
X33.-	Transfusion Blood Intravenous
X33.-	Transfusion Blood NEC
X34.1	Transfusion Coagulation Factor
X34.-	Transfusion Intravenous NEC
X32.-	Transfusion Plasma Exchange
X34.2	Transfusion Plasma NEC
X33.7	Transfusion Red Blood Cells Autologous
X33.7	Transfusion Red Blood Cells Perioperative
X33.7	Transfusion Red Blood Cells Post-operative
X32.6	Transfusion Red Cell Exchange
X34.3	Transfusion Serum NEC
	Translocation – see also Transfer
L41.5	Translocation Artery Renal Branch
C83.3	Translocation Macula Limited
C83.3	Translocation Macula NEC
C83.2	Translocation Macula Three Hundred & Sixty Degrees
V10.7	Translocation Orbit Subcranial
V10.6	Translocation Orbital
C83.-	Translocation Retina
C83.1	Translocation Retina Pigment Epithelium
	Transplantation – see also Allotransplantation
X04.1	Transplantation Adrenal Medulla to Brain Caudate Nucleus
X04.-	Transplantation Between Systems
W34.-	Transplantation Bone Marrow
C43.7	Transplantation Conjunctiva
C46.7	Transplantation Cornea Limbal Cells
J54.1	Transplantation Duodenum & Pancreas
T50.-	Transplantation Fascia
K01.-	Transplantation Heart & Lung
K01.2	Transplantation Heart & Lung Revision

K02.-	Transplantation Heart NEC
K02.4	Transplantation Heart Piggyback
K02.6	Transplantation Heart Revision NEC
G68.-	Transplantation Ileum
M01.-	Transplantation Kidney
M17.-	Transplantation Kidney Associated Interventions
J01.-	Transplantation Liver
J01.4	Transplantation Liver Cells
K01.-	Transplantation Lung & Heart
E53.1	Transplantation Lung Double
E53.-	Transplantation Lung NEC
E53.2	Transplantation Lung Single
E53.3	Transplantation Lung Single Lobe
T76.-	Transplantation Muscle
J54.-	Transplantation Pancreas
G68.-	Transplantation Small Intestine NEC
J72.1	Transplantation Spleen
X33.-	Transplantation Stem Cells Peripheral
G26.-	Transplantation Stomach
B17.-	Transplantation Thymus Gland
F08.-	Transplantation Tooth
	Transposition – see also Resiting
	Transposition – see also Translocation
K05.-	Transposition Arteries Great Operations Inversion Atrial
K48.2	Transposition Artery Coronary NEC
C35.1	Transposition Eye Muscle NEC
W77.7	Transposition Ligament NEC
C35.1	Transposition Muscle Eye NEC
W77.2	Transposition Muscle NEC
B35.1	Transposition Nipple
C08.1	Transposition Orbit Ligament
Q47.1	Transposition Ovary
B16.1	Transposition Parathyroid Tissue Modification
B14.8	Transposition Parathyroid Tissue NEC
F50.1	Transposition Parotid Duct
F50.-	Transposition Salivary Duct
F50.2	Transposition Submandibular Duct
T64.-	Transposition Tendon
L82.1	Transposition Vein Valve
C49.2	Trephine Cornea
C55.2	Trephine Corneoscleral
V03.5	Trephine Cranium
E14.6	Trephine Ethmoid Sinus
E14.6	Trephine Frontal Sinus
	Tube – see also Drainage
	Tube – see also Intubation
	Tube – see also Prosthesis
G08.-	Tube Oesophagus Feeding Open
G38.-	Tube Stomach Feeding Open
G44.7	Tube Stomach Removal Endoscopic Fibreoptic

G44.7	Tube Stomach Removal Endoscopic Fibreoptic Percutaneous
M49.-	Tube Suprapubic Attention
M38.2	Tube Suprapubic Insertion
D20.-	Tube Tympanic Membrane Ventilation Attention
D15.1	Tube Tympanic Membrane Ventilation Insertion
E95.-	Tuberculosis Support
	Tucking – see also Plication
C33.-	Tucking Eye Muscle
E04.-	Turbinate Operations
R07.-	Twin to Twin Operations Endoscopic
R08.-	Twin to Twin Operations Percutaneous
D14.-	Tympanoplasty
D14.4	Tympanoplasty Combined Approach
D15.-	Tympanotomy

U

Z71.-	Ulna site NEC
Y53.2	Ultrasonic Control Approach
U08.2	Ultrasound Abdomen NEC
U11.1	Ultrasound Artery Carotid
K51.2	Ultrasound Artery Coronary Intravascular
R42.3	Ultrasound Artery Fetus Cerebral Middle Doppler
L72.6	Ultrasound Artery Intravascular NEC
R42.1	Ultrasound Artery Umbilical Doppler
R42.2	Ultrasound Artery Uterine Doppler
M49.7	Ultrasound Bladder High Intensity Focused
U12.4	Ultrasound Bladder NEC
U13.2	Ultrasound Bone
	Ultrasound Examination – see also Examination
U13.2	Ultrasound Joint
U12.3	Ultrasound Kidneys
R43.-	Ultrasound Monitoring Pregnancy
U21.6	Ultrasound NEC
R42.-	Ultrasound Obstetric Doppler
U09.2	Ultrasound Pelvis NEC
M71.1	Ultrasound Prostate High Intensity Focused
C87.4	Ultrasound Retina
U12.2	Ultrasound Scrotum
U12.2	Ultrasound Testes
U06.3	Ultrasound Thyroid Gland
U35.3	Ultrasound Transcranial Doppler Velocimetry
Q55.5	Ultrasound Transvaginal
Q20.6	Ultrasound Uterus Lesion Focused
L98.6	Ultrasound Vessel Microvascular Anastomosis Doppler
U11.2	Ultrasound Vessels Extremities Doppler
T29.-	Umbilicus Operations
T29.6	Umbilicus Operations Plastic
Z53.2	Umbilicus site
T29.-	Umbilicus Skin Operations
Z53.2	Umbilicus Skin site
	Unblocking – see also Operation
L92.-	Unblocking Catheter Access
	Unfinished Operations – refer to Tabular List Introduction
L69.2	Unifocalisation Pulmonary
Z94.4	Unilateral Operations
	Unspecified Organ – see Organ Unspecified

M29.-	Ureter Operations Endoscopic Therapeutic NEC
M26.-	Ureter Operations Nephroscopic Therapeutic
M25.-	Ureter Operations Open NEC
M27.-	Ureter Operations Ureteroscopic Therapeutic
Z41.-	Ureter site
M18.-	Ureterectomy
M32.-	Ureteric Orifice Operations
M23.1	Ureterolithotomy Open
M25.3	Ureterolysis
M11.3	Ureterorenoscopy Diagnostic
M30.-	Ureteroscopy
M30.4	Ureteroscopy Nephroscopic
M19.-	Ureterostomy
M21.6	Ureteroureterostomy
M76.-	Urethra Operations Endoscopic Therapeutic
M79.-	Urethra Operations NEC
M75.-	Urethra Operations Open NEC
Z42.-	Urethra site
M81.-	Urethral Orifice Operations
M72.-	Urethrectomy
M72.4	Urethrectomy Secondary
M53.1	Urethrocleisis
M79.-	Urethrography
M52.4	Urethrolysis
M73.6	Urethroplasty NEC
M77.-	Urethroscopy
Y52.2	Urethrostomy Approach
M38.1	Urethrostomy Perineal & Drainage Bladder
M58.1	Urethrotomy Bladder Outlet Female Closed
M75.3	Urethrotomy External
M79.4	Urethrotomy Internal NEC
M76.3	Urethrotomy Optical
U26.3	Urinalysis Test Strip
M19.-	Urinary Diversion
M86.-	Urinary Diversion Operations Endoscopic Therapeutic
U26.-	Urinary System Diagnostic Testing
Z42.-	Urinary Tract Lower site
M83.-	Urinary Tract Operations NEC
Z41.-	Urinary Tract Upper site
U26.4	Urodynamics NEC
M47.4	Urodynamics Using Catheter
M48.2	Urodynamics Using Tube Suprapubic
U26.2	Uroflowmetry
X31.2	Urogram Intravenous
R30.-	Uterus Delivered Operations NEC
R12.-	Uterus Gravid Operations
Q52.-	Uterus Ligament Broad Operations
Z46.4	Uterus Ligament Broad site
Q54.-	Uterus Ligament Operations NEC
Q17.-	Uterus Operations Endoscopic Therapeutic

Q20.-	Uterus Operations NEC
Q09.-	Uterus Operations Open NEC
Q16.-	Uterus Operations Vaginal NEC
Z45.-	Uterus site NEC
F32.4	Uvula Operations NEC
F32.5	Uvulopalatopharyngoplasty
F32.6	Uvulopalatoplasty

V

E95.2	Vaccination Bacillus Calmette-Guerin
X44.-	Vaccination NEC
R22.-	Vacuum Delivery
P15.-	Vagina Introitus Operations NEC
P29.-	Vagina Operations NEC
P21.-	Vagina Operations Plastic
P32.-	Vagina Operations Plastic Other
Z44.-	Vagina site
Y50.3	Vaginal Approach
M53.-	Vaginal Operations Support Bladder Outlet Female NEC
M51.-	Vaginoabdominal Operations Support Bladder Outlet Female
Q20.4	Vaginofixation Uterus
P21.4	Vaginoplasty Absence Uterus & Vagina
P32.6	Vaginoplasty Mould & Skin Graft
P32.7	Vaginoplasty Mould NEC
P21.3	Vaginoplasty NEC
P21.5	Vaginoplasty Olive
P32.4	Vaginoplasty Rotational Skin Flaps
P32.5	Vaginoplasty Tissue Expanders
A27.-	Vagotomy NEC
K36.2	Valvectomy Pulmonary
K36.1	Valvectomy Tricuspid
K32.-	Valvotomy Closed
K31.-	Valvotomy NEC
K31.-	Valvotomy Open
K35.-	Valvotomy Transluminal Percutaneous
K26.5	Valvuloplasty Aortic NEC
K29.5	Valvuloplasty Heart NEC
K25.5	Valvuloplasty Mitral NEC
K28.5	Valvuloplasty Pulmonary NEC
K35.5	Valvuloplasty Transluminal Percutaneous
K27.6	Valvuloplasty Tricuspid NEC
K29.6	Valvuloplasty Truncal
N19.-	Varicocele Operations
L84.-	Varicose Vein Operations Primary Combined
L84.-	Varicose Vein Operations Recurrent Combined
Z40.6	Vascular Body site
Z40.-	Vascular Tissue site NEC
N17.-	Vasectomy
N18.-	Vasectomy Reversal

N20.5	Vasography
N20.4	Vasotomy
Z39.7	Vein Adrenal site
Z91.5	Vein Axillary site
Z91.3	Vein Brachial site
Z91.2	Vein Brachiocephalic site
Z91.1	Vein Cephalic site
Z98.-	Vein Femoral site
Y27.5	Vein Graft NOC
Z39.6	Vein Hepatic site
Z93.1	Vein Iliac site
Z98.-	Vein Lower Limb site NEC
L97.5	Vein Operations NEC
L93.-	Vein Operations Open NEC
L95.-	Vein Operations Transluminal Diagnostic
L94.-	Vein Operations Transluminal Therapeutic
L99.-	Vein Operations Transluminal Therapeutic Other
Z93.2	Vein Ovarian site
Z93.-	Vein Pelvis site NEC
Z98.4	Vein Popliteal site
Z39.3	Vein Portal site
L80.-	Vein Pulmonary Individual Operations
Z40.2	Vein Pulmonary site
L91.-	Vein Related Operations NEC
Z39.4	Vein Renal site
Z98.5	Vein Saphenous Long site
Z98.6	Vein Saphenous Short site
Z39.5	Vein Saphenous site NEC
Z39.-	Vein site NEC
Z91.4	Vein Subclavian site
Z93.3	Vein Testicular site
Z98.7	Vein Tibial site
Z91.-	Vein Upper Body site NEC
Z93.5	Vein Uterine site
L84.-	Vein Varicose Combined Operations Primary
L84.-	Vein Varicose Combined Operations Recurrent
L87.-	Vein Varicose Leg Operations NEC
G10.-	Vein Varicose Oesophagus Operations Open
U35.2	Velocimetry Laser Doppler Ultrasound
U35.3	Velocimetry Ultrasound Transcranial Doppler
L79.-	Vena Cava Operations NEC
Z39.-	Vena Cava site
X36.2	Venesection
L95.1	Venography NEC
J11.5	Venography Portal Intrahepatic Transjugular
L94.6	Venoplasty Transluminal Percutaneous
L83.-	Venous Insufficiency Operations NEC
X36.3	Venous Sampling
E85.4	Ventilation Bag Valve Mask
E85.3	Ventilation Improving Efficiency

E85.1	Ventilation Invasive
E85.5	Ventilation Nebuliser
E85.2	Ventilation Non-invasive NEC
E85.-	Ventilation Support
Z33.7	Ventricle Heart site
K24.-	Ventricles Heart Operations NEC
K24.-	Ventricular Outflow Tract Obstruction Operations
K23.5	Ventriculectomy Left Partial
A12.1	Ventriculocisternostomy
A20.2	Ventriculography Brain
A18.-	Ventriculoscopy Brain
A17.2	Ventriculostomy Third Endoscopic
R12.4	Version Cephalic External
Z66.-	Vertebra site
V44.4	Vertebroplasty Spine Fracture
N22.3	Vesiculography Seminal
L01.-	Vessel Great Abnormality Combined Operations Open
L03.-	Vessel Great Abnormality Operations Transluminal
D26.-	Vestibular Apparatus Operations
Z21.5	Vestibular Apparatus site
F11.4	Vestibuloplasty Mouth
Y53.6	Video Assisted Approach
Y74.4	Video Assisted Thoracoscopic Approach
C60.6	Viscocanulostomy
C61.5	Viscogonioplasty
C79.1	Vitrectomy Anterior Approach
C79.2	Vitrectomy NEC
C79.2	Vitrectomy Pars Plana Approach
C79.-	Vitreous Body Operations
Z19.2	Vitreous Body site
P09.-	Vulva Operations NEC
Z44.3	Vulva site
P09.-	Vulva Skin Operations NEC
Z44.3	Vulva Skin site
P05.-	Vulvectomy

W

S23.-	W Plasty
	Washout – see also Irrigation
B16.4	Washout Parathyroid
H42.-	Wiring Perianal Sphincter
W20.6	Wiring Sternum
X36.-	Withdrawal Blood
M17.3	Work-up Pre-transplantation Kidney Live Donor
M17.2	Work-up Pre-transplantation Kidney Recipient
	Wound – see Operation Skin
	Wound – see Operation Subcutaneous Tissue
O31.1	Wrist site NEC (Z)

X

U08.3	X-ray Abdomen Plain
U13.5	X-ray Bone Plain
U07.3	X-ray Chest Plain
U13.4	X-ray Joint Plain
U21.7	X-ray Plain NEC
U06.4	X-ray Skull Plain
Y27.3	Xenograft NOC
S37.-	Xenograft Skin
Y01.3	Xenoreplacement NOC
	Xenotransplantation – see Transplantation

Y

| X61.4 | Yoga |

Z

S23.-   Z Plasty

Section II

(D) = Device code assigned is the normal code for insertion or replacement.
Tabular List must be consulted for maintenance, removal etc.

Note: If the same operation can be done on different subsites e.g. parts of the spine, then the surgical eponym is assigned to the unspecified site and reference should be made to the Tabular List to identify the particular site.

A

F04.2	Abbe	Distant Flap Lip (Two Stage)
G61.1	Abbe	Jejunal Anastomosis Technique
F04.2	Abbe-Estlander	Local Pedicle Flap Cross Lip (One Stage)
X22.9	Adams	(D) Hip Pin Correction of Cong. Dislocation
W27.9	Adams	(D) Hip Pin for Fixation Epiphysis (Z76.1)
E03.8	Adams	Crushing Nasal Septum
W15.6	Akins	Cuneiform Osteotomy Proximal Phalanx
W31.2	Albee	Graft Tibia (Z77.2)
V38.3	Albee	Interspinous Fusion Lumbar Spine
X22.2	Albee	Osteotomy Pelvis
M52.1	Aldridge-Studdiford	Sling Urethral
H14.1	Allen-Welch	Caecostomy
G23.1	Allison	Repair Oesophageal Hiatus Hernia
D12.8	Almoor	Drainage Petrous Apex Mastoid
W40.-	Anametric	(D) Total Replacement Knee (Cemented)
W30.1	Anderson	(D) External Fixator
W17.2	Anderson	Leg Lengthening Procedure (Z90.9)
M05.1	Anderson-Hynes	Pyeloplasty
G24.6	Angelchick	(D) Prosthesis Antireflux Operation
D15.1	Armstrong	(D) Tube Ear
C54.4	Arruga	String Operation for Detached Retina
D26.8	Arslan	Fenestration Inner Ear
E43.1	Asai	Tracheo-oesophagoplasty
G11.-	Atkinson	(D) Prosthesis Oesophagus (Code to Procedure)
W40.-	Attenborough	(D) Total Replacement Knee (Cemented)
W37.-	Aufranc-Turner	(D) Total Replacement Hip (Cemented)
W46.-	Austin-Moore	(D) Hemiarthroplasty Hip (Cemented)
W47.-	Austin-Moore	(D) Hemiarthroplasty Hip (Uncemented)
D14.-	Austin-Shea	Myringoplasty
W40.-	Autophor	(D) Total Replacement Knee (Cemented)

B

L87.4	Babcock	Subcutaneous Enucleation Varicose Vein
M73.5	Badenoch	Pull Through Urethroplasty
V29.4	Badgeley	Anterior Fusion Cervical Spine
W60.1	Badgeley	Extra-articular Fusion Hip (Z84.3)
V29.4	Bailey	Anterior Fusion Cervical Spine
S20.1	Bakamjian	Flap Deltopectoral (Z49.9)
X25.1	Baker	Osteotomy Os Calcis
T70.3	Baker	Recession Gastrocnemius Muscle (Z58.1)
W31.3	Baldwin	Graft Wrist (Z70.4)
G29.2	Balfour	Excision Gastric Ulcer
G28.1	Balfour	Partial Gastrectomy
H49.8	Ball	Undercutting Perianal Skin
G01.1	Bancroft	Oesophagogastrectomy
W77.1	Bankart	Repair Shoulder (Z81.4)
V29.4	Barbour	Anterior Fusion Cervical Spine
C61.4	Barkan	Goniopuncture
C61.3	Barkan	Goniotomy
X49.1	Barlow	(D) Splintage for Cong. Disloc. Hip (Z90.2)
V46.4	Barr	(D) Skull Traction
T64.3	Barr	Ant. Transfer Tibialis Post. Tendon (Z58.3)
W61.1	Barr	Intra-articular Fusion Ankle (Z85.6)
H52.4	Barron	Band Haemorrhoidectomy
R21.3	Barton	Mid Forceps Rotation Fetal Head
P05.1	Bassett	Vulvectomy (T85)
T20.3	Bassini	Repair Inguinal Hernia
T21.3	Bassini	Repair Recurrent Inguinal Hernia
X48.1	Batchelor	(D) Plaster for Cong. Disloc.Hip (Z90.2)
W04.3	Batchelor	Subtalar Fusion
W57.2	Batchlor-Milch	Excision Arthroplasty Hip (Z84.3)
X09.4	Batch-Spittler-McFaddin	Disarticulation Knee
W47.-	Bateman	(D) Hemiarthroplasty Hip (Uncemented)
K23.5	Batista	Partial Left Ventriculectomy
W43.-	Beddow	(D) Total Replacement Shoulder (Cemented) (Z81.4)
J56.4	Beger	Subtotal Excision of Head of Pancreas
G24.1	Belsey	Antireflux Operation
W12.8	Benjamin	Double Osteotomy Knee (Z84.6)
X07.1	Berger	Interscapulothoracic Amputation Arm
Y82.1	Biers	Nerve Block IV
B31.1	Biesenberger	Reduction Breast
M44.1	Bigelow	Litholapaxy
G28.1	Billroth I	Partial Gastrectomy & Gastroduodenal Anastomosis
G28.3	Billroth II	Partial Gastrectomy & Gastroenterostomy
J07.8	Binnie	Hepatopexy
W58.-	Birmingham	(D) Resurfacing Arthroplasty of Hip (Z84.3)
M20.-	Bischoff	Replantation Ureter
K29.3	Bjork-Shiley	(D) Prosthesis Replacement Heart Valve NEC (Normally Code to Valve Replaced)
W61.1	Blair	Intra-articular Fusion Ankle (Z85.6)

K15.1	Blalock-Hanlon	Creation Defect Atrial Septum
L08.3	Blalock-Taussig	Anastomosis Subclavian to Pulmonary Artery
M73.4	Blandy	Reconstruction Urethra
C18.1	Blascovics	Resection Levator Muscle Eyelid
T20.3	Bloodgood	Repair Inguinal Hernia
T21.3	Bloodgood	Repair Recurrent Inguinal Hernia
W19.1	Blount	(D) Nail Plate Hip
W27.3	Blount	Staple Epiphysiodesis
M21.2	Boari	Creation Flap Bladder
J21.1	Bobb	Cholelithotomy
G05.-	Boerema	Button Anastomosis Oesophagus
W60.1	Bosworth	Extra-articular Fusion Hip (Z84.3)
X22.2	Bosworth	Osteotomy Pelvis
V38.2	Bosworth	Posterior Interlaminar Fusion Spine
W77.3	Bosworth	Repair Acromioclavicular Joint (Z81.2)
X10.2	Boyd	Amputation Hindfoot
X09.5	Boyd	Amputation Lower Leg
X23.2	Boyd	Bone Graft Pseudoarthrosis Tibia
X09.2	Boyd	Disarticulation Hip
M37.1	Bradford-Young	Cystourethroplasty
T64.2	Brand	Transfer Tendon Hand (Z56.9)
R30.2	Brandt-Andrews	Expression Placenta
M19.1	Bricker	Ileoureterostomy
E06.4	Brighton	Nasal Balloon Packing
W77.1	Bristow	Repair Shoulder (Z81.4)
W60.1	Brittain	Extra-articular Arthrodesis
W61.1	Brittain	Intra-articular Fusion Elbow (Z81.5)
W61.1	Brittain	Intra-articular Fusion Knee (Z84.6)
K32.4	Brock	Valvulotomy Pulmonary Valve
W59.3	Brockman	Fusion First Metatarsophalangeal Joint
G74.3	Brooke	Ileostomy
V37.-	Brooks	Fusion Atlantoaxial Joint
L91.1	Broviac	(D) Central Venous Catheter
X49.1	Browne(Denis)	(D) Splint for Club Foot (Z90.5)
M73.2	Browne(Denis)	Repair Epispadias
M73.1	Browne(Denis)	Repair Hypospadias
X49.1	Browne-Denis	(D) Splint for Club Foot (Z90.5)
M73.2	Browne-Denis	Repair Epispadias
M73.1	Browne-Denis	Repair Hypospadias
W19.4	Brown-Tulloch	(D) Sliding Nail Plate
V38.3	Buck	Fusion Spine for Spondylolisthesis
M52.3	Burch	Colposuspension
X09.5	Burgess	Amputation Lower Leg
M37.1	Burns	Cystourethroplasty
T25.1	Burton	Repair Incisional Hernia
X27.4	Butler	Soft Tissue Release Fifth Toe
M73.1	Byars	Repair Hypospadias

C

E12.2	Caldwell-Luc	Sublabial Drainage Maxillary Antrum
X09.4	Callander	Disarticulation Knee
W60.1	Campbell	Extra-articular Fusion Ankle (Z85.6)
T64.2	Campbell-Goldthwait	Transfer Patella Tendon (Z58.8)
K29.3	Carpentier-Edwards	(D) Prosthetic Replacement Heart Valve NEC (Normally Code to Valve Replaced)
C03.2	Castroviejo	(D) Eyeball Prosthesis
W43.-	Cavendish	(D) Total Replacement Elbow (Cemented) (Z81.5)
W40.9	Cavendish	(D) Total Replacement Knee (Cemented)
W43.-	Cavendish	(D) Total Replacement Shoulder (Cemented) (Z81.4)
M73.1	Cecil	Repair Hypospadias
G11.-	Celestin	(D) Prosthesis Oesophagus (Code to Procedure)
W60.1	Chandler	Extra-articular Fusion Hip (Z84.3)
T92.2	Charles	Correction Lymphoedema
W62.2	Charnley	(D) Compression Clamp for Fusion
W19.1	Charnley	(D) Compression Screw Hip
W37.-	Charnley	(D) Total Replacement Hip (Cemented)
W40.-	Charnley	(D) Total Replacement Knee (Cemented)
W62.2	Charnley	Compression Arthrodesis
W37.-	Charnley-Muller	(D) Total Replacement Hip (Cemented)
T22.3	Cheadle-Henry	Repair Femoral Hernia
T23.3	Cheadle-Henry	Repair Recurrent Femoral Hernia
X22.2	Chiari	Osteotomy Pelvis
J56.1	Childs	Pancreaticoduodenectomy
J57.1	Childs	Subtotal Pancreatectomy
W60.1	Cholmeley	Extra-articular Fusion Hip (Z84.3)
X10.4	Chopart	Midtarsal Amputation
T08.3	Clagett	Fenestration Chest Wall
V29.4	Cloward	Anterior Fusion Cervical Spine
L83.2	Cockett	Subfascial Ligation Perforating Varicose Vein
D26.8	Cody	Perforation Footplate
G24.5	Collis	Antireflux Operation
X22.3	Colonna	Arthroplasty Hip
W61.1	Coltart	Intra-articular Fusion Ankle (Z85.6)
F22.1	Commando	Glossectomy & Block Dissection (T85.1)
A12.4	Cordis-Hakim	(D) Valve Ventriculoperitoneal
W19.5	Coventry	(D) Cannulation Screw
X23.5	Coventry (MB)	Osteotomy Tibia
K52.6	Cox Maze	Incision Tissue Atria
X49.1	Craig	(D) Splintage for Cong. Disloc. Hip (Z90.2)
C18.3	Crawford	Tarsofrontalis Sling Eyelid Using Fascia
V46.4	Crutchfield	(D) Skull Traction
M05.1	Culp-Deweerd	Pyeloplasty
M05.1	Culp-Scardino	Pyeloplasty

D

C45.2	D'Ombrain	Excision Pterygium & Graft Cornea (C46.2)
G04.1	Dahlman	Excision Diverticulum Oesophagus
L06.2	Damus-Kaye-Stansel	Anastomosis Pulmonary Artery to Aorta
W08.5	Darrach	Distal Excision Ulna (Z71.6)
V21.8	Dautrey	Recurrent Temporomandibular Dislocation
P32.2	Davidov	Reconstruction Vagina Using Peritoneal Graft
M23.8	Davis	Ureterotomy Intubated
W40.-	Deane	(D) Total Replacement Knee (Cemented)
X19.9	Debeyre	Reconstruction Soft Tissue Shoulder
W43.-	Dee	(D) Total Replacement Elbow (Cemented) (Z81.5)
H41.1	Delorme	Excision Mucosa Rectum
K67.9	Delorme	Pericardiectomy
H36.8	Delorme	Repair Rectum for Prolapse
W29.9	Denham	(D) Bone Pin
W40.-	Denham	(D) Total Replacement Knee (Cemented)
X49.1	Denis-Browne	(D) Splint for Club Foot (Z90.5)
M73.1	Denis-Browne	Repair Hypospadias
E12.2	Denker	Radical Antrotomy Maxillary
	Denver	Shunt – see nature
D14.-	Derlacki	Myringoplasty
K34.2	De Vega	Annuloplasty Tricuspid Valve
H15.8	Devine	Colostomy
W19.1	Deyerle	(D) Pin Hip
X22.2	Dial	Osteotomy Pelvis
W03.3	Dickson-Diveley	Fusion Claw Toe with Transfer Tendon
X24.3	Dillwyn-Evans	Operation for Club Foot
E23.2	Dohlman	Repair Pharyngeal Pouch
	Dotter	Transluminal Angioplasty (Code to Vessel)
A27.1	Dragstedt	Subdiaphragmatic Truncal Vagotomy
M73.1	Duckett	Repair Hypospadias
H41.8	Duhamel	Incision Colorectal Septum
H41.8	Duhamel	Pull Through for Hirschsprung Disease
X49.1	Dunlop	(D) Traction System Arm (Z89.9)
W27.9	Dunn	(D) Hip Pin for Fixation Epiphysis (Z76.1)
W04.2	Dunn	Triple Fusion Foot
H36.8	Dunphy	Repair Rectum for Prolapse
X19.2	Durham	Operation for Erbs Palsy
T64.4	Durham-Caldwell	Transfer Biceps Femoris Tendon (Z57.6)
W77.3	Du Toit	Staple Capsulorrhaphy Shoulder (Z81.4)
J59.4	Duval	Pancreaticojejunostomy
V41.2	Dwyer	Anterior Wiring Spine for Scoliosis
T54.1	Dwyer (FC)	Fasciotomy
X25.1	Dwyer (FC)	Osteotomy Os Calcis

E

D12.8	Eagleton	Drainage Petrous Apex Mastoid
H53.8	Earle	Haemorrhoidectomy
L77.1	Eck	Side to Side Portocaval Shunt
W77.4	Eden-Hybinette	Block Bone for Recurrent Dislocation
W20.1	Eggers	(D) Fracture Plate
W78.3	Eggers (GWN)	Transfer Tendon Hamstring
C55.2	Elliot	Trephination Sclera
W20.1	Ellis	(D) Fracture Plate
W77.2	Ellison	Soft Tissue Repair Knee (Z84.6)
W77.2	Elmslie	Soft Tissue Stabilisation Ankle (Z85.6)
X25.2	Elmslie	Wedge Tarsectomy
T01.1	Eloesser	Thoracoplasty
W19.3	Ender	(D) Flexible Intramedullary Nail
H35.8	Erickman	Repair Rectum for Prolapse
W24.4	Essex-Lopresti	Operation for Fracture Os Calcis (Z79.2)
X24.3	Evans-Dillwyn	Operation for Club Foot
C18.1	Everbusch	Resection Levator Muscle Eyelid
W37.-	Exeter	(D) Total Replacement Hip (Cemented)

F

X19.2	Fairbank	Operation for Obstetric Palsy
C18.5	Fasanella-Servat	Tarsomullerectomy
P13.2	Fenton	Perineorrhaphy
T20.3	Ferguson	Repair Inguinal Hernia
T21.3	Ferguson	Repair Recurrent Inguinal Hernia
X22.1	Ferguson (AB)	Open Reduction Congenital Dislocation Hip
D26.8	Fick	Perforation Footplate
G40.3	Finney	Pyloroplasty
A27.2	Finney	Vagotomy & Pyloroplasty (G40.3)
W31.1	Fisk	Graft Scaphoid (Z72.2)
X09.2	Fitzmaurice-Kelly	Disarticulation Hip
L71.2	Fogarty	(D) Catheter Closed Embolectomy Artery (or Code to Artery)
L94.8	Fogarty	(D) Catheter Closed Embolectomy Vein (or Code to Vein)
M05.1	Foley	Pyeloplasty
K19.2	Fontan	Creation Conduit R.Atrium Pulmonary Artery
K18.2	Fontan	Creation Valved Conduit Right Atrium Pulmonary Artery
P22.2	Fothergill	Anterior Colporrhaphy & Amputation Cervix
D17.8	Fowler	Anterior Crurotomy
S70.1	Fowler	Avulsion Nail
W03.1	Fowler (AW)	Reconstruction Forefoot
W77.2	Fowler (SB)	Release Mallet Finger (Z83.5)
T64.1	Fowler (SB)	Transfer Muscle Forearm (Z55.9)
V33.3	Freebody	(D) Anterior Interbody Fusion Lumbar Spine
W37.-	Freeman	(D) Total Replacement Hip (Cemented)
W38.-	Freeman	(D) Total Replacement Hip (Uncemented)
W40.-	Freeman-Swanson	(D) Total Replacement Knee (Cemented)
X49.1	Frejka	(D) Splintage for Cong. Disloc. Hip (Z90.2)
D12.8	Frenckner	Drainage Petrous Apex Mastoid
M61.3	Freyer	Transvesical Prostatectomy
W37.-	Furlong	(D) Total Replacement Hip (Cemented)
W38.-	Furlong	(D) Total Replacement Hip (Uncemented)

G

H56.4	Gabriel	Excision Anal Fissure
H33.1	Gabriel	Resection Rectum
W77.2	Galeazzi	Tenodesis Semitendinosis Patellofemoral Joint (Z84.4)
T20.1	Gallie	Repair Inguinal Hernia Fascia Lata
T21.1	Gallie	Repair Recurrent Inguinal Hernia
W04.3	Gallie (WE)	Arthrodesis Subtalar Joint
V37.-	Gallie (WE)	Fusion Atlantoaxial Joint
T64.4	Garceau	Transfer Tibialis Anterior Muscle (Z58.4)
W24.1	Garden	(D) Cannulated Screw Hip
W12.9	Gariepy	Osteotomy Upper Tibia (Z77.1)
W40.-	Geomedic	(D) Total Replacement Knee (Cemented)
W40.-	Geometric	(D) Total Replacement Knee (Cemented)
W61.1	Ghormley	Intra-articular Fusion Hip (Z84.3)
H14.1	Gibson	Caecostomy
T92.4	Gibson-Tough	Correction Lymphoedema
W61.1	Gill (AB)	Intra-articular Fusion Shoulder (Z81.4)
X22.2	Gill (AB)	Osteotomy Pelvis
V43.-	Gill (GG)	Excision Spondylolisthesis
Q54.1	Gilliam	Suspension Uterus
V09.3	Gillies	Reduction Fracture Zygomatic Complex
W61.1	Gill-Stein	Intra-articular Fusion Wrist (Z82.1)
W57.2	Girdlestone	Excision Arthroplasty Hip (Z84.3)
T64.2	Girdlestone	Transfer Flexor Tendon Toe (Z59.2)
T64.4	Girdlestone	Transfer Pectoralis Major Tendon (Z54.3)
V27.1	Girdlestone (GR)	Laminectomy & Fusion Spine
T64.2	Girdlestone-Taylor	Transfer Flexor Tendon Toe (Z59.2)
W25.9	Gissane	(D) Spike Fixator
L09.1	Glenn	Anast. Superior Vena Cava R.Pulmonary Artery
W15.2	Golden	Osteotomy Base First Metatarsal Hallux Valgus
W04.3	Goldthwait	Stabilisation Hindfoot
W77.2	Goldthwait	Transfer Infrapatellar Tendon (Z84.4)
X09.1	Gordon-Taylor	Hindquarter Amputation
	Gortex	Prosthetic Material (Code to Procedure)
W04.3	Grice	Subtalar Fusion
X09.4	Gritti-Stokes	Disarticulation Knee
G74.8	Gross	Exteriorisation Operation Intestine
W19.2	Grosse-Kempf	(D) Intermedullary Nail Trochanter Femur (Z76.3)
X23.5	Gruca	Bifurcation Tibia
L71.5	Grunzig	(D) Catheter for Transluminal Dilation Artery (or Code to Artery)
W40.-	Guepar	(D) Total Replacement Knee (Cemented)
D17.1	Guildford	Stapedectomy
W40.-	Gunston	(D) Total Replacement Knee (Cemented)
X09.5	Guyon	Amputation Lower Leg

H

B34.1	Hadfield	Excision Subareolar Duct Breast
W27.8	Hagie	(D) Hip Pin for Fixation Epiphysis (Z76.1)
A12.4	Hakim	Insertion Ventriculoperitoneal Shunt
A12.2	Halber	(D) Valve for Spina Bifida
B27.1	Halsted	Mastectomy (T85.2)
T20.8	Halsted	Repair Inguinal Hernia
T21.3	Halsted	Repair Recurrent Inguinal Hernia
L23.2	Hamilton	Flap Repair Coarctation Aorta
M05.1	Hamilton-Stewart	Pyeloplasty & Plication Kidney (M05.4)
H05.1	Hampton	Ileorectal Anastomosis
V41.1	Harrington	(D) Instrumentation Spine
V46.2	Harrington	(D) Rod Fixation Fracture Spine
W62.-	Harrison Nicholle	(D) Prosthetic Peg for Joint Fusion
H33.5	Hartmann	Resection Rectum
V41.1	Hartshill	(D) Instrumentation Spine
W46.-	Hastings	(D) Hemiarthroplasty Hip (Cemented)
T64.4	Hauser	Transfer Infrapatellar Tendon (Z57.3)
E95.1	Heaf	Tuberculosis test
Q08.9	Heaney	Vaginal Hysterectomy
G40.3	Heinecke-Mickulicz	Pyloroplasty
A27.2	Heinecke-Mikulicz	Vagotomy & Pyloroplasty (G40.3)
W56.-	Helal	(D) Arthroplasty Metatarsophalangeal Joint
W03.2	Helal	Osteotomy Metatarsal Bone
G09.1	Heller	Cardiomyotomy
L41.5	Hellstrom	Translocation Renal Vessel
M43.2	Helmstein	Prolonged Hydrostatic Overdistension Bladder
C19.8	Henderson	Incision Muller Muscle Eyelid
W61.1	Henderson (MS)	Intra-articular Fusion Hip (Z84.3)
W19.5	Herbert	(D) Small Fragment Screw
W40.-	Herbert	(D) Total Replacement Knee (Cemented)
X10.9	Hey	Amputation Foot
W74.2	Hey-Groves	Reconstruction Ant.Cruciate Ligament (Z84.6)
W27.2	Heymann-Herndon	Clearance Joint (Z76.1)
W03.8	Heymann-Herndon	Correction Metatarsus Varus
V38.2	Hibbs	Fusion Lumbar Spine
W61.1	Hibbs	Intra-articular Fusion Hip (Z84.3)
L91.1	Hickman	(D) Central Venous Catheter
W20.1	Hicks	(D) Fracture Plate
G24.4	Hill	Gastropexy Antireflux Operation
T64.4	Hitchcock	Transposition Biceps Brachii (Z54.4)
W30.1	Hoffmann	(D) External Fixator
G28.3	Hofmeister	Valved Gastrectomy
W15.1	Hohmann	Osteotomy Neck First Metatarsal Hallux Valgus
W04.2	Hoke	Fusion Hindfoot
W19.1	Holt	(D) Nail Hip
A20.1	Holter	(D) Valve Drainage Ventricle
T92.4	Homan	Correction Lymphoedema
E14.4	Horgan	Transantral Ethmoidectomy
D17.1	Hough	Stapedectomy
D17.1	House	Stapedectomy

E14.1	Howarth	External Frontoethmoidectomy
W37.-	Howse	(D) Total Replacement Hip (Cemented)
T64.2	Huber	Transfer Thenar Muscle (Z56.2)
W19.2	Huckster	(D) Intermedullary Nail & Screw
M20.-	Hutch	Replantation Ureter
E21.1	Hynes	Pharyngoplasty
M05.1	Hynes-Anderson	Pyeloplasty

I

W58.-	Ilch	(D) Surface Replacement Hip (Z84.3)
W37.-	Ilch	(D) Total Replacement Hip (Cemented)
W40.-	Ilch	(D) Total Replacement Knee (Cemented)
X49.1	Ilfield	(D) Splintage for Cong. Disloc. Hip (Z90.2)
W43.-	Irving	(D) Total Replacement Ankle (Cemented) (Z85.6)
W40.-	Irving	(D) Total Replacement Knee (Cemented)
T83.2	Irwin	Myotomy
	Ivalon	Sponge Prosthetic Material (Code to Procedure)
G01.1	Ivor-Lewis	Oesophagogastrectomy

J

N11.3	Jaboulay	Eversion Hydrocele Sac
X09.1	Jaboulay	Hindquarter Amputation
G31.3	Jabouley	Gastroduodenostomy
A32.4	Janetta	Microvascular Decompression Facial Nerve
E14.4	Jansen-Horgan	Transantral Ethmoidectomy
C35.1	Jensen	Transposition Muscles Eye
W19.1	Jewett	(D) Nail Plate Hip
M73.4	Johanson	Reconstruction Urethra
C25.1	Jones	Canaliculodacryocystorhinostomy
Q09.5	Jones	Metroplasty
T67.8	Jones	Repair Peroneal Tendon (Z58.2)
W74.2	Jones (KG)	Reconstruction Ant. Cruciate Ligament (Z84.6)
W57.2	Jones (L)	Resection Head Humerus (Z69.1)
W03.3	Jones (R)	Operation for Claw Toe
W03.4	Jones (R)	Transfer Tendon to First Metatarsal
W12.2	Jones (R)	Valgus Osteotomy Hip (Z76.2)
W60.1	Jones (W)	Extra-articular Fusion Shoulder (Z81.4)
W61.1	Jones (W)	Intra-articular Fusion Hip (Z84.3)
W77.2	Jones (W)	Stabilisation Ankle (Z85.6)
T64.4	Joplin	Sling Procedure Muscle Foot (Z59.-)
W79.1	Joplin	Soft Tissue Operation for Hallux Valgus
X19.1	Josserand	Scapulopexy
W47.-	Judet	(D) Hemiarthroplasty Hip (Uncemented)
T64.4	Judet	Pedicle Graft Gluteus Muscle (Z57.1)
T79.2	Judet	Quadricepsplasty

K

J29.1	Kasai	Hepatojejunostomy
W03.1	Kates-Kessel	Reconstruction Forefoot
M75.2	Kaufman	(D) Prosthesis Male Incontinence
T25.3	Keel	Repair Incisional Hernia
N08.3	Keetley-Torek	Bilateral Orchidopexy First Stage
N08.4	Keetley-Torek	Bilateral Orchidopexy Second Stage
N09.3	Keetley-Torek	Unilateral Orchidopexy First Stage
N09.4	Keetley-Torek	Unilateral Orchidopexy Second Stage
J07.8	Kehr	Hepatopexy
W32.1	Keil	(D) Prepared Graft Bone
W57.1	Keller	Excision Arthroplasty First MTP Joint
M53.1	Kelly-Kennedy	Urethrovesical Plication
W43.-	Kessel	(D) Total Replacement Shoulder (Cemented) (Z81.4)
W03.1	Kessel-Kates	Reconstruction Forefoot
W61.1	Key	Intra-articular Fusion Knee (Z84.6)
R21.3	Kielland	Mid Forceps Rotation Fetal Head
E14.1	Killian	External Frontoethmoidectomy
F29.1	Kilner-Wardill	Repair Cleft Palate
X09.1	King-Steelquist	Hindquarter Amputation
X09.3	Kirk	Amputation Thigh
X09.4	Kirk	Disarticulation Knee
W29.1	Kirschner	(D) Wire Fixation
J72.4	Kirschner	Repair of Spleen
V41.1	Knodt	(D) Spinal Distraction Rod
G74.1	Koch	Continent Ileostomy
T92.8	Kondoleon	Correction Lymphoedema
K37.6	Konno	Aortoventriculoplasty
A75.9	Krause	Sympathetic Denervation
C06.9	Kroenlein	Lateral Orbitotomy
X07.5	Krukenberg	Amputation Below Elbow
C15.1	Kuhnt-Szymanowski	Repair Ectropion
W19.2	Kuntschner	(D) Intramedullary Fixation
S22.4	Kutler	Local Flap Closure Finger Tip (Z50.3)

L

G53.6	Ladd	Correction Malrotation Duodenum
W04.2	Lambrinudi	Triple Fusion Joints Hindfoot
F29.1	Langenbeck	Repair Cleft Palate
W59.3	Lapidus	Arthrodesis M.T.P. Joint for Hallux Valgus
T71.1	Lapidus	Synovectomy Peroneal Tendon (Z58.2)
X27.4	Lapidus	Transplantation Tendon Fifth Toe
X07.2	Larry	Disarticulation Shoulder
P18.2	Latzko	Partial Colpocleisis
M73.4	Leadbetter	Reconstruction Urethra
M19.2	Leadbetter	Ureterosigmoidostomy
M20.-	Leadbetter-Politano	Replantation Ureter
K06.2	Lecompte	Direct Ventriculo-arterial Connection
P18.1	Le Fort	Complete Colpocleisis
V10.4	Le Fort	Osteotomy Maxilla
F03.1	Lemesurier	Repair Cleft Lip
A75.4	Leriche	Perivascular Sympathectomy
C25.3	Lester-Jones	(D) Dacryocystorhinostomy Tube
L81.1	Le Veen	(D) Peritoneovenous Shunt
S27.-	Limberg	Random Pattern Local Flap Skin
W74.1	Lindemann	Muscle Transfer Knee (Z84.6)
T67.9	Lindholm	Repair Rupture Tendon
W54.-	Link	Arthroplasty Joint
L87.8	Linton	Interruption Perforating Varicose Vein
L83.2	Linton	Subfacial Ligation Perforating Vein Leg
T64.4	Lippman	Transportation Biceps Brachii (Z54.4)
T72.3	Lipscomb-Duvries	Tenosynoplasty Peroneal Tendon (Z58.2)
X07.2	Lisfranc	Disarticulation Shoulder
X10.3	Lisfranc	Tarsometatarsal Amputation
X07.1	Littlewood	Forequarter Amputation
W40.-	Liverpool	(D) Total Replacement Knee (Cemented)
H33.1	Lloyd-Davis	Resection Rectum
H51.1	Lockhart-Mummery	Haemorrhoidectomy
T22.3	Lockwood	Repair Femoral Hernia
T23.3	Lockwood	Repair Recurrent Femoral Hernia
J29.-	Longmire	Biliary Bypass
W38.-	Lord	(D) Total Replacement Hip (Uncemented)
N11.2	Lord	Plication Hydrocele Sac
W12.2	Lorenz	Osteotomy Hip (Z76.2)
T23.3	Lotheissen	Repair Recurrent Femoral Hernia
T22.3	Lothiessen	Repair Femoral Hernia
W19.3	Lottes	(D) Intramedullary Nail Tibia (Z77.2)
W77.8	Lowman	Transfer Tendon Tibialis Anterior (Z86.2)
W55.-	Luck	(D) Interposit. Cup Arthroplasty Hip (Z84.3)
E14.1	Luc-Ogston	External Frontoethmoidectomy
X22.1	Ludloff	Open Reduction Congenital Dislocation Hip
V41.1	Luque	(D) Instrumentation Spine

M

W55.-	Macintosh	(D) Plateau Prosthesis Tibia Knee (Z84.6)
W77.2	Macintosh	Plastic Stabilisation Tenodesis Knee (Z84.6)
W38.-	Madreporique	(D) Total Replacement Hip (Uncemented)
W77.2	Magnuson-Stack	Op. for Recur. Dislocation Shoulder (Z81.3)
T25.3	Maingot	Repair Incisional Hernia
G28.8	Maki	Partial Gastrectomy Preserving Pylorus
T20.2	Maloney	(D) Nylon Darn Repair Inguinal Hernia
T21.2	Maloney	Repair Recurrent Inguinal Hernia
W40.-	Manchester	(D) Total Replacement Knee (Cemented)
P22.9	Manchester	Colporrhaphy
T70.3	Maquet	Elevation Tubercle Tibia (Z57.3)
W40.-	Marmor	(D) Total Replacement Knee (Cemented)
M52.2	Marshall-Marchetti-Krantz	Retropubic Suspension Urethra
G30.2	Mason	Gastric Partitioning
G23.1	Mason	Repair Oesophageal Hiatus Hernia
W19.1	Massie	(D) Nail Plate Hip
W47.-	Matchett-Brown	(D) Hemiarthroplasty Hip (Uncemented)
W31.1	Mattie-Russe	Graft Scaphoid (Z72.2)
H41.8	Maunsell-Weir	Proctectomy
W43.-	Mayo	(D) Total Replacement Elbow (Cemented) (Z81.5)
H35.4	Mayo	Repair Rectum for Prolapse
T24.3	Mayo	Repair Umbilical Hernia
L87.3	Mayo	Stripping Varicose Vein
W57.1	Mayo (CH)	Excision Arthroplasty First MTP Joint
G33.1	Mayo-Ward	Gastroenterostomy
X09.4	Mazet	Disarticulation Knee
W20.1	McAtee	(D) Fixation Olecranon (Z71.1)
W79.1	McBride	Soft Tissue Operation for Hallux Valgus
P23.4	McCall	Repair Enterocele
V20.9	McCarthy	Arthroplasty Temporomandibular Joint
R12.1	McDonald	Encirclement Suture Cervix Gravid Uterus
T22.3	McEvedy	Repair Femoral Hernia
T23.3	McEvedy	Repair Recurrent Femoral Hernia
X23.2	McFarland	Bone Graft Pseudoarthrosis Tibia
D16.8	McGee	Malleostapediopexy
P21.1	McIndoe	Construction Vagina
T52.1	McIndoe (A)	Fasciectomy Palm
W40.-	McKee	(D) Total Replacement Knee (Cemented)
W37.-	McKee-Farrer	(D) Total Replacement Hip (Cemented)
G02.2	McKeown	Oesophagectomy
B31.1	McKssock	Reduction Breast
W19.1	McLaughlin	(D) Nail Plate Hip
W77.1	McLaughlin	Repair Shoulder (Z81.3)
W13.3	McMurray	Osteotomy Hip (Z76.2)
T20.3	McVay	Repair Inguinal Hernia
T21.3	Mcvay	Repair Recurrent Inguinal Hernia
W40.-	Melbourne	(D) Total Replacement Knee (Cemented)
J05.3	Menghini	(D) Biopsy Liver (Open)
J13.2	Menghini	(D) Biopsy Liver (Percutaneous)
S42.-	Michel	(D) Clip Skin Closure

W57.2	Milch-Batchelor	Excision Arthroplasty Hip (Z84.3)
H33.1	Miles	Resection Rectum
F03.1	Millard	Repair Cleft Lip
W03.8	Miller	Fusion Midtarsus
H51.1	Milligan-Morgan	Haemorrhoidectomy
M61.2	Millin	Retropubic Prostatectomy
M52.1	Millin-Reed	Suspension Urethrovesical
W37.-	Minneapolis	(D) Total Replacement Hip (Cemented)
W38.-	Minneapolis	(D) Total Replacement Hip (Uncemented)
H53.8	Mitchell	Haemorrhoidectomy
W15.1	Mitchell	Osteotomy Neck First Metatarsal Hallux Valgus
M19.2	Mitrofanoff	Urinary Diversion
V38.-	Moe	Posterior Joint Fusion Spine
S05.-	Mohs	Chemosurgical Excision Skin
C60.5	Molteno	(D) Implantation Tube Anterior Chamber Eye
W46.-	Monk	(D) Hemiarthroplasty Hip (Cemented)
W47.-	Monk	(D) Hemiarthroplasty Hip (Uncemented)
W37.-	Monk	(D) Total Replacement Hip (Cemented)
W38.-	Monk	(D) Total Replacement Hip (Uncemented)
W27.9	Moore	(D) Hip Pin for Fixation Epiphysis (Z76.1)
W46.-	Moore-Austin	(D) Hemiarthroplasty Hip (Cemented)
K24.6	Morrow	Left Ventricular Myectomy & Myotomy
P23.4	Moschowitz	Repair Enterocele
H19.8	Moschowitz	Sigmoid Colonopexy (Z28.6)
G28.3	Moynihan-Mayo	Partial Gastrectomy
W43.-	Mueli	(D) Total Replacement Wrist (Cemented) (Z82.1)
W37.-	Muller	(D) Total Replacement Hip (Cemented)
K05.-	Mustard	Reconstruction Transposition Great Arteries
T64.4	Mustard	Transplant Iliopsoas (Z57.2)
C11.3	Mustarde	Canthoplasty for Correction Epicanthus
D03.3	Mustarde	Pinnaplasty

N

A47.1	Nashold	Needling Substantia Gelatinosa Cervical Reg.
W49.-	Neer	(D) Hemiarthroplasty Shoulder (Cemented)
W50.-	Neer	(D) Hemiarthroplasty Shoulder (Uncemented)
N28.3	Nesbitt	Plication Corpora of Penis
W19.1	Neufield	(D) Nail Plate Hip
W77.1	Neviaser	Repair Shoulder (Z81.2)
W77.2	Nicola	Tenodesis Shoulder (Z81.4)
W01.3	Nicolandi	Osteoplastic Reconstruction Thumb
W45.-	Nicolle	(D) Total Replacement MCP Joint (Z83.2)
W55.-	Niebauer	(D) Prosthetic Replacement MCP Joint (Z83.-)
G24.3	Nissen	Abdominal Antireflux Operation
G24.1	Nissen	Thoracic Antireflux Operation
G76.4	Noble	Plication Intestine
K17.3	Norwood	Aortopulmonary Reconstruction Procedure
	Nottingham	(D) Prosthesis Oesophagus (Code to Procedure)
T25.3	Nuttall	Repair Incisional Hernia

O

W75.1	O'Donoghue	Repair Ligament Knee (Z84.6)
W78.2	O'Malley	Release Capsule Hip for Osteoarthritis
W77.2	Ober	Operation for Recur. Disloc. Patella (Z84.4)
T55.3	Ober-Yount	Gluteoiliotibial Fasciotomy
V16.2	Obwegeser	Osteotomy of Mandible
F11.4	Obwegeser	Vestibuloplasty Mouth
N08.2	Ombredanne	Bilateral Orchidopexy One Stage
M73.1	Ombredanne	Repair Hypospadias
N09.2	Ombredanne	Unilateral Orchidopexy One Stage
E21.3	Orticochea	Pharyngoplasty
T64.4	Osmond-Clark	Transfer Peroneus Brevis Tendon (Z58.2)
M79.4	Otis	Internal Urethrotomy
W30.1	Oxford	(D) External Fixator

P

T70.3	Page	Muscle Slide Forearm (Z55.1)
L83.1	Palma	Cross Over Saphenous Graft
Q55.-	Papanicolau	Cervical Smear
M20.-	Paquin	Replantation Ureter
W20.2	Parham	(D) Cerclage Band
H04.2	Parks	Creation Ileal Pouch
H51.8	Parks	Submucosal Haemorrhoidectomy
B27.3	Patey	Mastectomy (T85.2)
D08.2	Pattee	Reconstruction External Auditory Canal
H15.-	Paul-Mickulicz	Colostomy
H10.5	Paul-Mickulicz	Resection Colon
W12.9	Pauwels	Osteotomy Upper Femur (Z76.2)
X49.1	Pavlik	(D) Splintage for Cong. Disloc. Hip (Z90.2)
G61.3	Payne-Dewind	Jejunocolostomy
X49.1	Pearson	(D) Splint Knee (Z84.6)
A75.5	Peet	Resection Splanchnic Nerve
X22.2	Pemberton	Osteotomy Ilium
M51.2	Pereyra	Endoscopic Suspension Bladder Neck
X49.1	Perkins	(D) Traction System Leg (Z90.-)
X24.3	Perkins	Operation for Club Foot
D15.1	Perlee	(D) Tube Ear
J59.3	Peustow	Pancreaticojejunostomy
M53.8	Peyera-Raz-Gitter	Colposuspension Vaginal
W31.9	Phemister	Bone Graft
W27.1	Phemister	Epiphysiodesis
X10.1	Pirogoff	Amputation Ankle
W40.-	Platt	(D) Total Replacement Knee (Cemented)
M20.-	Politano-Leadbetter	Replantation Ureter
G28.3	Polya	Partial Gastrectomy
W40.-	Polycentric	(D) Total Replacement Knee (Cemented)
Q27.1	Pomeroy	Bilateral Ligation Fallopian Tubes
T70.5	Poncet	Lengthening Tendo Achillis (Z58.1)
W91.2	Ponsetti Treatment	Manipulation Joint (Z86.9)
D16.8	Portman	Malleostapediopexy
L06.4	Potts-Smith	Anast. Descending Aorta L. Pulmonary Artery
W37.-	Pretoria	(D) Total Replacement Hip (Cemented)
W40.-	Pretoria	(D) Total Replacement Knee (Cemented)
W71.3	Pridie	Forage Knee (Z84.6)
G33.1	Printer-Mason	Gastroenterostomy
W43.-	Pritchard-Walker	(D) Total Replacement Elbow (Cemented) (Z81.5)
W19.1	Pugh	(D) Nail Plate Hip
X49.1	Pugh	(D) Traction System
W60.1	Putti	Intra-articular Fusion
W77.1	Putti-Platt	Repair Shoulder (Z81.3)

R

D12.8	Ramadier	Drainage Petrous Apex Mastoid
G40.1	Rammstedt	Pyloromyotomy
H11.9	Rankin	Colectomy
H33.1	Rankin	Resection Rectum
V22.8	Ransford	Decompression Cervical Spine
K16.1	Rashkind	Balloon Atrial Septostomy
K18.3	Rastelli	Creation Valved Conduit Pulmonary Artery
W62.2	Ratliff	Compression Fusion Ankle (Z85.6)
X08.4	Ray	Amputation of Finger
X10.4	Ray	Transmetatarsal Amputation
K06.2	Rev	Direct Ventriculo-arterial Connection
W19.1	Richards	(D) Screw Hip
W38.-	Ring	(D) Total Replacement Hip (Uncemented)
X20.3	Riordan	Operation for Congenital Absence Radius
W01.5	Riordan	Transfer Opponens Thumb
H35.4	Ripstein	Repair Rectum for Prolapse NEC
H35.2	Ripstein	Repair Rectum for Prolapse Using Teflon
V29.4	Robinson-Smith	Discectomy & Fusion Cervical Spine
J57.1	Rodney-Smith	Distal Pancreatectomy
J29.1	Rodney-Smith	Hepatojejunostomy
J56.2	Rodney-Smith	Pancreaticoduodenectomy
W06.8	Roos	Excision First Rib (Z74.3)
H36.1	Roscoe-Graham	Repair Rectum for Prolapse
M75.2	Rosen	(D) Prosthesis Male Incontinence
K33.1	Ross	Pulmonary Autograft Aortic Root Replacement
W19.1	Ross-Brown	(D) Nail Hip
K33.2	Ross-Konno	Aortoventriculoplasty Pulmonary Autograft
M10.4	Rosving	Deroofing of Multiple Cysts of Kidney
J19.3	Roux-en-Y	Cholecystojejunostomy
J30.2	Roux-en-Y	Choledochojejunostomy
G01.2	Roux-en-Y	Oesophagogastrectomy
J59.-	Roux-en-Y	Pancreaticojejunostomy
W77.2	Roux-Goldthwaite	Stabilisation Knee By Transplant. Tendon (Z84.4)
G02.3	Roux-Herzen-Judine	Oesophagectomy
X27.4	Ruiz-Mora	Excision Proximal Phalanx Fifth Toe
W19.3	Rush	(D) Intramedullary Nail
X49.1	Russell-Hamilton	(D) Traction System Leg (Z90.9)

S

X22.2	Salter	Osteotomy Pelvis
J29.1	Sawaguchi	Hepatojejunostomy
W12.2	Schanz	Osteotomy Hip (Z76.2)
Q08.-	Schauta	Radical Vaginal Hysterectomy – refer to Tabular List Introduction
T01.1	Schede	Thoracoplasty
C55.8	Scheie	Cautery Incision Sclera
G27.-	Schlatter	Total Gastrectomy
W19.2	Schnieder	(D) Nail for Forearm Fracture (Z71.3)
P14.1	Schuchardt	Episiotomy Non Obstetrical
D16.8	Schuknecht	Malleostapediopexy
D10.3	Schwartze	Cortical Mastoidectomy
T64.1	Schwarzmann-Crego	Transfer Hamstring (Z57.7)
G61.3	Scott	Jejunocolostomy
T64.8	Seddon-Brooks	Transfer Pectoralis Major Tendon (Z54.3)
L72.1	Seldinger	Arteriography (Or Code to Artery)
G21.-	Sengstaken	(D) Intubation Oesophagus
G21.-	Sengstaken-Blakemore	(D) Intubation Oesophagus
K05.-	Senning	Reconstruction Transposition Great Arteries
X19.2	Sever	Operation for Erbs Palsy
W77.2	Sharrard	Transfer Iliopsoas Muscle (Z57.2)
D16.8	Shea	Malleostapediopexy
D16.8	Shea-Guilford	Malleostapediopexy
J05.3	Sheeba	(D) Biopsy Liver (Open)
J13.2	Sheeba	(D) Biopsy Liver (Percutaneous)
W40.-	Sheehan	(D) Total Replacement Knee (Cemented)
W40.-	Shiers	(D) Total Replacement Knee (Cemented)
R12.1	Shirodkar	Encirclement Suture Cervix Gravid Uterus
Q05.1	Shirodkar	Repair Internal Os Cervix Uteri
T20.3	Shouldice	Repair Inguinal Hernia
T21.3	Shouldice	Repair Recurrent Inguinal Hernia
W79.2	Silver	Bunionectomy
T70.3	Silver	Recession Gastrocnemius Muscle (Z58.1)
T70.3	Silverskoild	Recession Gastrocnemius Muscle (Z58.1)
D15.1	Silverstein	(D) Tube Ear
B10.1	Sistrunk	Excision Thyroglossal Cyst
X09.4	Slocum	Disarticulation Knee
W77.2	Slocum	Transfer Pes Anserinus (Z84.6)
W21.3	Smillie	(D) Intra-articular Fragment Pin
W55.-	Smith-Petersen	(D) Interposition Arthroplasty
W62.1	Smith-Petersen	Intra-articular Fusion Hip (Z84.3)
W24.1	Smith-Petersen (M)	(D) Nail Hip
A75.1	Smithwick	Cervical Sympathectomy
H41.8	Soave	Operation for Hirschsprung Disease
W16.1	Sofield	Multiple Osteotomy & Fixation
W13.1	Somerville	Rotation Osteotomy Femur (Z76.3)
X09.1	Sorondo-Ferre	Hindquarter Amputation
W13.3	Southwick	Osteotomy Femur (Z76.2)
G11.-	Souttar	(D) Prosthesis Oesophagus (Code to Procedure)
W78.2	Soutter	Soft Tissue Release Hip

X07.2	Spence	Disarticulation Shoulder
M58.8	Spence	Vaginal Urethrocystostomy
D10.1	Stacke	Radical Mastoidectomy
M51.2	Stamey	Endoscopic Suspension Bladder Neck
W13.2	Stamm	Osteotomy Glenoid (Z68.4)
W37.-	Stanmore	(D) Total Replacement Hip (Cemented)
W40.-	Stanmore	(D) Total Replacement Knee (Cemented)
W43.-	Stanmore	(D) Total Replacement Shoulder (Cemented) (Z81.4)
W61.1	Staples	Intra-articular Fusion Elbow (Z81.5)
X20.3	Starr	Operation for Congenital Absence Radius
K29.3	Starr-Edwards	(D) Caged Prosthetic Replacement Heart Valve NEC (Normally Code to Valve Replaced)
X22.2	Steez	Osteotomy Pelvis
T54.2	Steindler	Release Plantar Fascia
W61.1	Steindler (A)	Intra-articular Fusion Elbow (Z81.5)
W61.1	Steindler (A)	Intra-articular Fusion Shoulder (Z81.4)
T64.1	Steindler (A)	Transfer Flexor Muscle Forearm (Z55.1)
W29.9	Steinmann	(D) Traction System
M05.1	Stewart-Hamilton	Pyeloplasty & Plication Kidney (M05.4)
W58.-	St Georg	(D) Resurfacing Arthroplasty Knee (Z84.6)
H51.1	St Mark	Haemorrhoidectomy
H33.1	St Mark	Resection Rectum
H50.9	Stone	Anoplasty
Q09.5	Strassman	Metroplasty
T70.5	Strayer	Recession Gastrocnemius Muscle (Z58.1)
B31.1	Strombeck	Reduction Breast
J05.8	Stromeyer-Little	Hepatotomy
Q03.1	Sturmdorf	Conisation Cervix Uteri
G60.1	Surmay	Jejunostomy Operation
X22.2	Sutherland	Osteotomy Pelvis
K65.2	Swan-Ganz	(D) Catheter Heart
W54.-	Swanson	Arthroplasty Joint
H41.8	Swenson	Operation for Hirschsprung Disease
T24.3	Swenson	Repair Umbilical Hernia
X10.1	Syme	Amputation Ankle
M75.3	Syme	External Urethrotomy

T

T36.8	Talma-Morison	Omentopexy
M73.4	Tanagho	Reconstruction Urethra
G10.8	Tanner	Gastric Transection
T20.3	Tanner	Repair Inguinal Hernia
T21.3	Tanner	Repair Recurrent Inguinal Hernia
F03.1	Tenison-Randall	Repair Cleft Lip
G24.5	Thal	Stricturoplasty Antireflux Operation
G24.5	Thal-Nissen	Stricturoplasty Antireflux Operation
W58.-	Tharies	(D) Resurfacing Replacement Hip (Z84.3)
S35.-	Thiersch	Split Autograft Skin
H42.1	Thiersch	Wire for Prolapse Rectum
X40.1	Thomas	(D) Intravascular Shunt for Dialysis
X49.1	Thomas	(D) Splint Leg (Z90.9)
T92.3	Thompson	Correction Lymphoedema
W46.-	Thompson (Fr)	(D) Hemiarthroplasty Hip (Cemented)
W47.-	Thompson (FR)	(D) Hemiarthroplasty Hip (Uncemented)
T79.2	Thompson (TC)	Quadricepsplasty
J18.5	Thorek	Partial Cholecystectomy
W19.1	Thornton	(D) Nail Plate Hip
O10.-	Tikhoff Linberg	Complex Reconstruction of Shoulder (W)
Q09.5	Tompkins	Metroplasty
N08.2	Torek-Bevan	Bilateral Orchidopexy One Stage
N09.2	Torek-Bevan	Unilateral Orchidopexy One Stage
A12.1	Torkildsen	Ventriculocisternostomy
L38.2	Touroff	Ligation Subclavian Artery
L85.1	Trendelenburg	High Ligation Long Saphenous Vein
L12.4	Trendelenburg	Pulmonary Embolectomy
W60.1	Trumble	Extra-articular Fusion Hip (Z84.3)
X24.1	Turco	Soft Tissue Release for Club Foot
M73.4	Turner-Warwick	Reconstruction Urethra

U

| W40.- | Uci | (D) Total Replacement Knee (Cemented) |

V

Q10.8	Vabra Aspiration	Biopsy Endometrium
M73.1	Van Der Meulen	Repair Hypospadias
X23.6	Vannes	Rotationplasty Leg
P21.5	Vecchietti	Construction of Vagina
F11.3	Visor-Sandwich	Augmentation Alveolar Ridge
L88.2	VNUS Closure	Radiofrequency Ablation of Varicose Vein of Leg
X49.1	Von Rosen	(D) Splintage for Cong. Disloc. Hip (Z90.2)
W78.2	Voss	Release Capsule Hip for Osteoarthritis
T70.5	Vulpius	Elongation Tendo Achillis (Z58.1)

W

W30.1	Wagner	(D) External Fixator
W17.2	Wagner	(D) Lengthening Leg (Z90.9)
W58.-	Wagner	(D) Surface Replacement Hip (Z84.3)
W40.-	Walldius	(D) Hinge Arthroplasty Knee (Cemented)
F29.1	Wardill	Repair Cleft Palate
L81.2	Waterhouse	Glanscorpora Shunt for Priapism
L06.3	Waterston	Anastomosis Aorta to Right Pulmonary Artery
W77.2	Watson-Jones	Tenodesis Stabilisation Ankle (Z58.2)
T67.9	Watson-Jones	Tenoplasty
W61.1	Watson-Jones (R)	Intra-articular Fusion Ankle (Z85.6)
W77.1	Weaver & Dunn	Repair Shoulder (Z81.2)
H14.8	Weir	Appendicostomy
E02.8	Weir	Correction Nostril
H35.2	Wells	Repair Rectum for Prolapse
Q07.-	Wertheim	Radical Hysterectomy – refer to Tabular List Introduction
T64.9	Westminster	Relocation Tendon
C15.2	Wheeler	Repair Entropion
J56.2	Whipple	Pancreaticoduodenectomy
T70.5	White	Lengthening Tendo Achillis (Z58.1)
H51.1	Whitehead	Haemorrhoidectomy
T79.8	Whitman	Repair Serratus Anterior Muscle (Z60.8)
W06.8	Whitman	Talectomy (Z79.1)
F50.1	Wilke	Bilateral Diversion Parotid Duct
P21.1	Williams	Construction Vagina
T01.1	Wilms	Thoracoplasty
W15.1	Wilson	Osteotomy Neck First Metatarsal Hallux Valgus
V38.3	Wiltse	Posterior Fusion Lumbar Spine
J19.4	Winiwater	Cholecystoenterostomy
L81.2	Winter	Glanscorpora Shunt for Priapism
G75.-	Witzel	Temporary Enterostomy
S36.-	Wolfe	Full Thickness Skin Graft
U40.2	Wood's light	Diagnostic Ultraviolet Skin Test
X19.1	Woodward	Reconstruction Soft Tissue Shoulder
D14.-	Wullstein	Myringoplasty

Y

H40.2	York-Mason	Excision Lesion Rectum
H40.8	York-Mason	Repair Fistula Rectum
M73.1	Young	Repair Hypospadias
T64.9	Young	Transfer Tendon
M73.2	Young-Dees	Repair Epispadias
W78.3	Yount	Soft Tissue Release Knee

Z

Section III

Alphabetical Index
of
Surgical Abbreviations

Code	Abbreviation	Description
W71.4	ACI	Autologous Cartilage Implantation
M55.6	ACT	Adjustable Continence Therapy
X09.3	AKA	Above Knee Amputation
O19.1	AMIC	Autologous Matrix Induced Chondrogenesis (W)
H33.1	AP	Abdominoperineal Resection Rectum
D13.-	BAHA	Bone Anchored Hearing Aid
E13.6	BAWO	Bilateral Antral Washout
E95.2	BCG	Bacillus Calmette-Guerin Vaccination
X09.5	BKA	Below Knee Amputation
W34.-	BMT	Bone Marrow Transplant
E85.2	BPAP	Bilevel Positive Airway Pressure
E85.2	CNP	Continuous Negative Airway Pressure
E85.2	CPAP	Continuous Positive Airway Pressure
U21.2	CT	Computed Axial Tomography Scanning
Y94.1	DATSCAN	Dopamine Transporter Scan
C25.-	DCR	Dacryocystorhinostomy
U13.1	DEXA	Dual Emission X-Ray Absorptiometry Scan
W24.2	DHS	Dynamic Hip Screw Closed
W24.1	DHS	Dynamic Hip Screw Closed Intracapsular
W19.1	DHS	Dynamic Hip Screw Open
B39.3	DIEP	Deep Inferior Epigastric Perforator Flap
L06.2	DKS	Anastomosis Pulmonary Artery to Aorta
Y94.4	DTPA	Diethylenetriamine Pentacetic Acid Imaging
E63.2	EBUS-TBNA	Endobronchial Ultrasound Guided Transbronchial Needle Aspiration
X58.1	ECMO	Extracorporeal Membrane Oxygenation
A83.-	ECT	Electroconvulsive Therapy
R12.4	ECV	External Cephalic Version
M10.5	ENDOBRST	Endoscopic Endoluminal Balloon Rupture Stenosis Pelviureteric Junction Kidney
M27.6	ENDOBRST	Endoscopic Endoluminal Balloon Rupture Stenosis Ureter
L27.-	EVAR	Endovascular Aneurysm Repair
L88.1	EVLT	Endovascular Laser Therapy of Saphenous Varicose Vein
L88.3	EVLT	Endovascular Laser Therapy of Varicose Vein NEC
O11.1	GOJ	Gastro-oesophageal Junction site (Z)
M49.7	HIFU	High Intensity Focused Ultrasound Bladder
M71.1	HIFU	High Intensity Focused Ultrasound Prostate
K59.-	ICD	Implantable Cardioverter Defibrillator
Y96.-	ICIS	Intracytoplasmic Injection of Sperm
B38.2	IGAP	Inferior Gluteal Artery Perforator Flap
Q13.1	IVF	In Vitro Fertilisation
L72.6	IVUS	Intravascular Ultrasound Artery
K51.2	IVUS	Intravascular Ultrasound Coronary Artery

Code	Abbreviation	Description
C44.5	LASEK	Laser Subepithelial Keratomileusis
C44.2	LASIK	Laser in Situ Keratomileusis
U12.6	MAG3	Mercaptoacetyltriglycine Renogram
L69.-	MAPCAs	Major Systemic to Pulmonary Collateral Arteries
N34.4	MESA	Microsurgical Epididymal Sperm Aspiration
Y94.3	MIBG	Metaiodobenzylguanidine Imaging
U16.2	MRCP	Magnetic Resonance Cholangiopancreatography
U21.1	MRI	Magnetic Resonance Imaging Scanning NEC
U10.7	MUGA	Multiple Gated Acquisition Scan
E85.2	NIPPV	Non-Invasive Positive Pressure Ventilation
U21.1	NMR	Nuclear Magnetic Resonance Scanning NEC
E98.-	NRT	Nicotine Replacement Therapy
W83.7	OATS	Osteoarticular Transfer System
E91.3	ODI	Oxygen Desaturation Index Measurement
H41.2	PART	Peranal Resection Tumour
X33.-	PBSCT	Peripheral Blood Stem Cell Transplant
H15.7	PEC	Percutaneous Endoscopic Sigmoid Colostomy
E93.1	PEF	Peak Expiratory Flow Rate Study
G44.5	PEG	Percutaneous Endoscopic Gastrostomy
N34.5	PESA	Percutaneous Epididymal Sperm Aspiration
U21.3	PET	Positron Emission Tomography
L99.7	PICC	Percutaneous Transluminal Insertion Central Catheter
C44.4	PRK	Photorefractive Keratectomy
J77.1	PTVS	Percutaneous Transhepatic Portal Venous Sampling
O29.1	SAD	Subacromial Decompression (Open) (W)
U17.2	SeHCAT	Selenium-75-Homocholic Acid Taurine Study
B38.1	SGAP	Superior Gluteal Artery Perforator Flap
J12.3	SIRT	Selective Internal Radiotherapy with Microspheres Lesion Liver
W84.7	SLAP	Superior Labrum Anterior Posterior Repair
U21.4	SPECT	Single Photon Emission Computed Tomography
U28.-	SST	Serum Skin Test
U29.7	SST	Short Synacthen Test
H41.5	STARR	Stapled Transanal Rectal Resection
Q11.-	STOP	Suction Termination of Pregnancy
X65.1	TBI	Total Body Irradiation
A70.7	TENS	Transcutaneous Electrical Nerve Stimulator
N34.6	TESE	Testicular Sperm Extraction
J11.4	TIPS	Transjugular Intrahepatic Portosystemic Shunt
U20.2	TOE	Transoesophageal Echocardiography
M53.6	TOT	Introduction Transobtruator Tape
B39.-	TRAM	Transverse Rectus Abdominis Myocutaneous Flap
U20.1	TTE	Transthoracic Echocardiography
R07.-	TTTS	Twin to Twin Transfusion Syndrome
R08.-	TTTS	Twin to Twin Transfusion Syndrome

Code	Abbreviation	Description
Q48.1	TUDOR	Transurethral Ultrasound Directed Oocyte Recovery
M70.7	TUNA	Transurethral Radiofrequency Needle Ablation
M65.-	TURP	Transurethral Resection Prostate
M53.3	TVT	Introduction Tension-Free Vaginal Tape
F32.6	UVP	Uvulopalatoplasty
F32.5	UVPP	Uvulopalatopharyngoplasty
Y74.4	VATS	Video-Assisted Thoracoscopic Surgery
U15.3	VQ	Ventilation Perfusion Quotient Scan

Section IV

Alphabetical Index
of
Common Surgical Suffixes

Suffix	Meaning
anastomosis	Connection
-centesis	Puncture
-clasis	Fracture
-cleisis	Shutting In
-clysis	Rectal Injection
-desis	Binding
dialysis	Cleaning
	Compensation
-ectasia	Dilation
	Fusion
	Stabilisation
	Stretching
-ectomy	Excision
-exeresis	Removal
	Stripping Off
-graphy	Visual Display
-lysis	Freeing from Adhesions
	Loosening
-ostomy	Opening
-otomy	Incision
	Opening
-paxy	Crushing
	Washout
-pexy	Fixing
	Suspension
-plasty	Moulding
	Reformation
-plexy	Weaving
-rrhaphy	Suturing
-schisis	Division
-scopy	Inspection
-stasis	Positioning
	Stopping
-stomy	Making A Mouth
	Opening
-tasis	Stretching
-taxis	Arranging
-tome	Cutting Instrument
-tomy	Cutting (Not Puncture)
	Section
-tripsy	Crushing
-trity	Crushing